Provided as a service by Boehringer Ingelheim Pharmaceuticals, Inc., distributor of ATROVENT® (ipratropium bromide) Inhalation Solution and ATROVENT® (ipratropium bromide) Inhalation Aerosol.

Product Information:

The ususal dose of ATROVENT® (ipratropium bromide) Inhalation Solution is 500 mcg (1 unit-dose vial) administered 3 to 4 times a day, with doses 6 to 8 hours apart, by oral nebulization at settings recommended by the manufacturer.

ATROVENT® Inhalation Solution 0.02% Unit-dose Vials contain 500 mcg ATROVENT® diluted with normal saline to a total volume of 2.5 ml.

ATROVENT® Inhalation Solution Unit-dose Vial is supplied as a 0.02% clear, colorless solution containing 2.5 ml with 25 vials per foil pouch.

AS-5493R

Emergency Medicine Handbook

*Detroit Receiving Hospital
and University Health Center*

Third edition

Editor
William A. Berk, M.D.
Assistant Professor
Department of Emergency Medicine
Wayne State University School of Medicine
Attending Physician, Emergency Department
Detroit Receiving Hospital and University Health Center

Contributing Editors
Padraic J. Sweeny, M.D.
Assistant Professor
Department of Emergency Medicine
Wayne State University School of Medicine
Vice-Chief, Emergency Department
Detroit Receiving Hospital and University Health Center

Christopher J. Heberer, M.D.
Assistant Professor
Department of Emergency Medicine
Wayne State University School of Medicine
Attending Physician, Emergency Department
Detroit Receiving Hospital and University Health Center

Judith C. Andersen, M.D.
Associate Professor
Department of Internal Medicine
Wayne State University School of Medicine
Attending Physician, Department of Internal Medicine
Detroit Receiving Hospital and University Health Center

Plymouth Press
Plymouth, Michigan

ISBN 1-882663-01-2

1 2 3 4 5 6 7 8 9 10

Cover drawing of Detroit Receiving Hospital by Keith Brown.

Preface to third edition

The *Handbook* was conceived as a means of compiling the information most frequently used—but not memorized—by emergency physicians in a format easy to use and carry.

The *Handbook* is a collaboration of the faculty of the Department of Emergency Medicine at Wayne State University School of Medicine and Detroit Receiving Hospital/University Health Center. Section editors are:

Drug Therapy	Robert Wahl, M.D.
	Robert Welch, M.D.
	Robert Malinowski, M.D.
	David B. Levy, Pharm. D., A.E.M.T.
Trauma	Brooks F. Bock, M.D.
Toxicology	Suzanne White, M.D.
	Jim Cisek, M.D.
Critical Care	Robert Welch, M.D.
Pediatric Reference	Joseph Kosnik, M.D.

Gail M. Stewart, D.O. served as pediatric consultant editor.

There were many others who made significant contributions to this third edition. Jonathan Sullivan, M.D. contributed the drawing on page 120, and Steve Yucht, M.D. had the idea for and researched the information depicted on page 118. Anthony Achille, R.Ph; Violet Geisz, R.Ph.; Elizabeth Lyons, Pharm. D.; David "D.J." Stimac, R.Ph.; Elizabeth Raphael, M.D.; Evan Leibner, M.D.; and John Bair, M.D. helped verify the accuracy of drug doses. D.J. Stimac, R.Ph. and Elizabeth Lyons, Pharm. D. coordinated data collection for the table on prices of outpatient medications. Leon Levy of West Coast Pharmacy in San Francisco also contributed information for this table. Ross Tabbey, M.D., was kind enough to review the ACLS protocols for completeness and accuracy. Pattie Peterson, M.D. reviewed and corrected data for the figure on p. 120.

Administrative support was provided by Kathleen Barker, P.A.-C. and Pam Nelson. Keir Todd, P.A.-C. organized the business aspects of the *Handbook*. Once again, Brooks Bock, M.D. provided encouragement as well as material support during the months of work on this edition.

Every effort was made to ensure the accuracy of the contents of the *Handbook*. All drug doses were obtained from authoritative sources, but should be verified prior to being used to treat patients. Medicine is a constantly changing discipline and readers should keep in mind that all treatment recommendations are meant as guidelines subject to revision by medical authorities.

William A. Berk, M.D.

Contents

ECG interpretation aids .... *Inside front cover*
Visual acuity chart .... *Inside back cover*

Drug Therapy   1
  Drug Therapy in Pregnancy 1
  Drug Therapy of Specific Disease Entities 6
  Pediatric and Adult Drug Dosing 36
  Prescription Eye Medications 105
  Prices of Oral Outpatient Medications 106

Diagnostic Aids   111
  Dental Anatomy 111
  Hand Sensory Nerve Innervation 111
  Hand Motor Exam 112
  Hand Muscles by Nerve Innervation 114
  Spinal Cord Levels Sensory and Motor 115
  Sensory Dermatomes 116
  Cervical Spine Radiologic Parameters 118
  Cervical Spine Injuries: Stable and Unstable 119
  Coma: Correlating Exam Findings with Level
      of Brain Dysfunction 120

Toxicology   121
  General Protocol for Ingestions 121
  Protocol for Cutaneous Decontamination 122
  Protocol for Tricyclic Antidepressant Ingestion 123
  Osmolality Formulae 123
  Salicylate Overdose Nomogram 124
  Acetaminophen Overdose Nomogram 125

Toxidromes 126
Treatable by Hemodialysis or Hemoperfusion 127
Antidotes to Specific Overdoses 128
Phone Resources for Toxicologic Information 132

Trauma   133

Tetanus Wound Prophylaxis 133
Revised Adult Trauma Score 134
Adult Glasgow Coma Scale 135
Pediatric Trauma Score 136
Pediatric Coma Scale 137
Burn Surface Area 138
Rabies Prophylaxis 140

Critical Care   141

ACLS Protocols 141
Ventricular Fibrillation/Pulseless Ventricular
  Tachycardia 141
Asystole 142
Pulseless electrical activity 143
Wide Complex Tachycardia of Uncertain Origin 144
Sustained Ventricular Tachycardia with a Pulse 145
Polymorphic Ventricular Tachycardia 146
Symptomatic Bradycardia 147
Atrial Fibrillation or Flutter with
  Rapid Ventricular Rate 148
Narrow QRS Complex Tachycardia (PSVT) 149
Rapid Sequence Intubation Protocol 150
Dobutamine Dosing Table 152
Dopamine Dosing Table 153
Esmolol Dosing Table 154
Nitroprusside Dosing Table 155
Cardiovascular Formulae 156
Normal Resting Hemodynamic Values 158

General Medicine 159

Intravenous Fluid Components 159
Causes of Metabolic Acidosis 160
Causes of Metabolic Alkalosis 161
Acid-Base Nomogram 162
Acid-Base Assessment Formulae 163
Acute Renal Failure vs. Pre-Renal Azotemia 164
Body Surface Area Nomogram 165
Pediatric Normal Peak Expiratory Flow 166
Adult Normal Peak Expiratory Flow 167
Hemophilia A and B Treatment 168
Von Willebrand's Disease Treatment 170
Catheter Clearance Protocol 171
Isolation Strategies and Contagious Periods
    for Infectious Diseases 172
Synovial Fluid in Acute Arthritis 174

Pediatric Reference 175

Immunization Schedule 175
APGAR Scoring 176
Tube and Laryngoscope Sizes 176
Vital Signs by Age 177
Hematologic Indices by Age 177
Hemoglobin and MCV by Age 178
Normal Blood Pressure by Age 179
Girls' Weight and Length Birth to 36 Months 180
Boys' Weight and Length Birth to 36 Months 181
Girls' Weight and Height 2 to 18 Years 182
Boys' Weight and Height 2 to 18 Years 183
Girls' Head Circumference 184
Boys' Head Circumference 185

Index 186

1
Drug Therapy

See index for generic names of proprietary meds

In Pregnancy

Avoid unnecessary medication during pregnancy.

1 = safe in pregnancy for all accepted indications.
2 = accepted for some conditions, but may adversely affect fetus or other
    meds usually preferred for some indications—further reference advised.
3 = few if any indications during pregnancy.
* = avoid in first trimester.
† = avoid in third trimester.

Acebutolol 2	Amitriptyline 2	Beclomethasone 2
Acetaminophen 1	Amlodipine 2	Benazepril 3
Acetaminophen/	Amoxapine 2	Benztropine
codeine 2*	Amoxicillin 1	mesylate 2
Acetazolamide 2	Amoxicillin/	Bepridil 2
Acetohexamide 3	clavulanate 1	Betaxolol 2
Acetylcysteine 2	Ampicillin 1	Bethanecol 2
Acyclovir 2	Ampicillin/	Bicarbonate 2
Adenosine 2	sulbactam 1	Bitolterol 2
Albumin 1	Anistreplase 2	Bisacodyl 2
Albuterol 1	Antipyrine/	Bisoprolol fumarate 2
Allopurinol 2	benzocaine 2	Bretylium 2
Alprazolam 2*	Aspirin .... 2†	Bumetanide 2
Alteplase 2	Astemizole .... 2†	Buspirone 2
Aluminum	Atenolol 2	Butoconazole 2
hydroxide 1	Atovaquone 2	Butorphanol 2
Amantidine 2	Atracurium 2	Calcitriol 2
Amikacin 2	Atropine 2	Calcium chloride 2
Amiloride 2	Azithromycin 2	Calcium gluconate 2
Aminophylline 1	Aztreonam 2	Capsaicin 2
Amiodarone 2	Baclofen 2	Captopril 3

In Pregnancy   *See index for generic names of proprietary meds*

1 = safe in pregnancy for all accepted indications.
2 = accepted for some conditions, but may adversely affect fetus or other
    meds usually preferred for some indications—further reference advised.

Carbamazepine 2	Chlorpropamide 3	Diflunisal ....2†
Carbenicillin 1	Chlorthalidone 2	Digoxin 2
Carisoprodol 3	Chlorzoxazone 2	Digoxin immune
Carteolol 3	Cholestyramine 2	FAB 2
Cefaclor 1	Cimetidine 1	Dihydroergotamine
Cefadroxil 1	Cinoxacin 3	mesylate 3
Cefamandole 1	Ciprofloxacin 3	Diltiazem 2
Cefazolin 1	Cisapride 2	Dimenhydrinate 3
Cefixime 1	Clarithromycin 3	Diphenhydramine 1*
Cefmetazole 1	Clindamycin 1	Diphenoxylate/
Cefonicid 1	Clonazepam 2	atropine 1
Cefoperazone 1	Clonidine 2	Dipyridamole 2
Cefotaxime 1	Clorazepate 2*	Disopyramide 2
Cefotetan 1	Clotrimazole 1	Disulfiram 2
Cefoxitin 1	Cloxacillin 1	Dobutamine 2
Cefpodoxime 1	Codeine 2*	Docusate sodium 2
Cefprozil 1	Colchicine 3	Dopamine 2
Ceftazidime 1	Colestipol 2	Doxacurium
Ceftizoxime 1	Cromolyn sodium ... 1	chloride 2
Ceftriaxone 1	Crotamiton 2	Doxazosin 2
Cefuroxime 1	Cyclobenzaprine 2	Doxepin 2
Cephalexin 1	Cyproheptadine 2	Doxycycline 3
Cephalothin 1	Dapsone 2	Eflornithine 2
Cephapirin 1	Deferoxamine 2	Enalapril 3
Cephradine 1	Dexamethasone 2	Enoxacin 3
Chloral hydrate 2	Dextromethorphan 1	Epinephrine 2
Chloramphenicol .... 2†	Dextrose 1	Epinephrine,
Chlordiazepoxide ... 2*	Diazepam 2	racemic 2
Chlordiazepoxide/	Dichlorphenamide 2	Ergotamine 3
clidinium 2*	Diclofenac ....2†	Ergotamine/
Chlorothiazide 2	Dicloxacillin 1	caffeine 3
Chlorpheniramine .. 2	Dicyclomine 2	Erythromycin
Chlorpromazine 2	Didanosine 2	base 1

See index for generic names of proprietary meds   **In Pregnancy**

3 = few if any indications during pregnancy.
* = avoid in first trimester.
† = avoid in third trimester.

Erythromycin estolate 1	Furazolidone 2	Indomethacin .... 2†
Erythromycin ethylsuccinate 1	Furosemide 2	Insulin 1
	Ganciclovir 2	Ipratropium bromide 1
Erythromycin lactobionate or gluceptate 1	Gemfibrozil 2	Isoetharine 1
	Gentamicin 2	Isoniazid 1
	Glipizide 3	Isoproterenol 1
Erythromycin stearate 1	Glucagon 2	Isosorbide dinitrate 2
Erythromycin/ sulfisoxazole .... 2†	Glyburide 3	Isradipine 2
	Glycerin 2	Itraconazole 2
Esmolol 2	Glycopyrrolate 2	*Kayexalate* 1
Ethambutol 1	Griseofulvin 3	Ketamine .... 2†
Ethionamide 2	Guanabenz 2	Ketoconazole 2
Ethosuximide 1	Guanfacine 2	Ketoprofen .... 2†
Etodolac .... 2†	Haloperidol 2	Ketorolac .... 2†
Famotidine 1	Heparin 1	Labetalol 2
Felodipine 2	Hepatitis B immune globulin 1	Lactulose 1
Fenoprofen .... 2†		Laudanum 3
Fentanyl 2	Hepatitis B vaccine 2	Levothyroxine 1
Ferrous fumarate 1	Hydralazine 2	Lidocaine 2
Ferrous gluconate ... 1	Hydrochloro- thiazide 2	Lindane 3
Ferrous sulfate 1		Liothyronine 1
Flavoxate 2	Hydrochlorothiazide/ spironolactone 2	Lisinopril 3
Flecainide 2		Lithium 2*
Fluconazole 2	Hydrochlorothiazide/ triamterene 2	Lomefloxacin 3
Flucytosine 2		Loperamide 3
Flunisolide 2	Hydrocodone/ acetaminophen 2*	Loratadine 2
Fluoxetine 2		Lorazepam 2*
Fluphenazine 2	Hydrocortisone 2	Lovastatin 3
Flurbiprofen .... 2†	Ibuprofen .... 2†	Loxapine 2
Folic acid 1	Imipenem/ cilastatin 2	Magnesium citrate 2
Fosinopril 3	Imipramine 2	
	Indapamide 2	

In Pregnancy   *See index for generic names of proprietary meds*

1 = safe in pregnancy for all accepted indications.
2 = accepted for some conditions, but may adversely affect fetus or other
    meds usually preferred for some indications—further reference advised.

Magnesium sulfate ... 1	Mexilitene ... 2	Omeprazole ... 2
Mannitol ... 2	Mezlocillin ... 2	Opium tincture ... 3
Maprotiline ... 2	Miconazole ... 1	Orphenadrine ... 2
Mebendazole ... 3	Midazolam ... 2	Orphenadrine/ aspirin/caffeine ... 3
Meclizine ... 2	Minocycline ... 3	
Meclofenamate ... 2†	Minoxidil ... 3	Oxacillin ... 1
Mefenamic acid ... 2†	Misoprostol ... 3	Oxaprozin ... 2†
Meperidine ... 2	Morphine sulfate ... 2	Oxybutynin ... 2
Metaproterenol ... 1	Mupirocin ... 2	Oxycodone ... 2*
Methadone ... 2	Nabumetone ... 2†	Oxycodone/ acetaminophen ... 2*
Methazolamide ... 2	Nadolol ... 2	
Methenamine hippurate ... 2	Nafcillin ... 1	Oxycodone/ aspirin ... 2*†
	Nalbuphine ... 2	
Methenamine mandelate ... 2	Nalidixic acid ... 3	Pancuronium ... 2
	Naloxone ... 1	Paregoric ... 3
Methenamine phenylsalicylate/ atropine/ hyoscyamine ... 3	Naproxen ... 2†	Paroxetine ... 2
	Neomycin ... 2	Penicillin ... 1
	Neostigmine ... 2	Pentamidine ... 2
	Netilmicin ... 2	Pentazocine ... 2
Methicillin ... 1	Nicardipine ... 2	Pentobarbital ... 2
Methimazole ... 3	Niclosamide ... 2	Pentoxifylline ... 2
Methocarbamol ... 2	Nicotine transdermal ... 2	Permethrin ... 1
Methsuximide ... 3		Perphenazine ... 2
Methychlothiazide 2	Nifedipine ... 2	Phenazopyridine ... 2
Methyldopa ... 1	Nimodipine ... 2	Phenelzine ... 2
Methylene blue ... 2	Nitrofurantoin ... 1†	Phenobarbital ... 2
Methysergide ... 3	Nitroglycerin ... 2	Phenylbutazone ... 2†
Metoclopramide ... 1	Nitroprusside ... 3	Phenytoin ... 2
Metocurine iodide ... 2	Nizatidine ... 1	Pindolol ... 2
Metolazone ... 2	Norfloxacin ... 3	Piperacillin ... 1
Metoprolol ... 2	Nortriptyline ... 2	Pirbuterol ... 1
Metronidazole ... 2*	Nystatin ... 1	Piroxicam ... 2†
	Ofloxacin ... 3	Polyethylene glycol 2

See index for generic names of proprietary meds

In Pregnancy

3 = few if any indications during pregnancy.
* = avoid in first trimester.
† = avoid in third trimester.

Pralidoxime 1	Salsalate .... 2†	Thiethylperazine 3
Pravastatin 3	Scopolamine 2	Thioridazine 2
Prazosin 2	Selenium sulfide 2	Thiothixene 2
Primidone 2	Sertraline 2	Ticarcillin 1
Probenecid 1	Simethicone 1	Ticarcillin
Probucol 2	Simvastatin 3	clavulanate 1
Procainamide 2	Sodium polystyrene	Timolol 2
Prochlorperazine .... 2†	sulfonate 1	Tioconazole 1
Promethazine 2	Sotalol 2	Tobramycin 2
Propafenone 2	Spectinomycin 1	Tocainide 2
Propoxyphene 2	Spironolactone 2	Tolazamide 3
Propoxyphene/	Streptokinase 2*	Tolbutamide 3
acetaminophen 2	Succinylcholine 2	Tolmetin .... 2†
Propranolol 2	Sucralfate 1	Trancylpromine 2*
Protamine sulfate 2	Sulfadiazine .... 2†	Triamcinolone
Pseudoephedrine 2	Sulfadiazine, silver 2†	inhaler 2
Pyrantel pamoate 2	Sulfadoxine/	Triamterene 2
Pyrazinamide 2	pyrimethamine 2	Triazolam 3
Pyrethrins/piperonyl	Sulfamethoxazole ... 2†	Trifluoperazine 2
butoxide *(RID)* 2	Sulfasalazine .... 2†	Trimethadione 3
Pyrimethamine 2	Sulfisoxazole .... 2†	Trimethobenz-
Quinacrine 2	Sulindac .... 2†	amide 2
Quinapril 3	Sumatriptan 2	Trimethoprim 2
Quinidine gluconate 2	Terazosin 2	Trimethoprim/
Quinidine poly-	Terbinafine 2	sulfa .... 2†
galacturonate 2	Terbutaline 1	Valproic acid 3
Quinidine sulfate 2	Terconazole 2	Vancomycin 2
Quinine 2	Terfenadine 2	Vecuronium 2
Ramipril 3	Tetanus immune	Verapamil 2
Ranitidine 1	globulin 1	Vitamin K 2
Ribavirin 3	Tetanus toxoid 1	Warfarin 3
Rifampin 2	Tetracycline 3	Zalcitabine 2
Rimantadine 2	Thiabendazole 2	Zidovudine 2

Drug Therapy of Specific Disease Entities   *For generic names of proprietary meds, see index*

DISEASE	REGIMEN
Adrenal insufficiency	After drawing serum cortisol and ACTH levels: hydrocortisone 100 mg IV bolus, then *either* 10 mg/h infusion *or* 100 mg IV Q6h . Replace sodium/water deficits.
Alcohol withdrawal	[D5/NS 500-1000 ml with MgSO4 4 g *and* thiamine 100 mg IV over 1h *and either* (phenobarbital 260 mg IV over 20min *or* lorazepam 2-4 mg IV *or* diazepam 3-5 mg IV)]. Subsequent doses of phenobarbital 130 mg IV Q30min *or* lorazepam 1-3 mg IV *or* diazepam 3-5 mg IV to achieve light sedation.
Anaphylactic shock	[(Epinephrine 1:1000 0.01 ml/kg *(child)* or 0.2-0.5 mg *(adult)* IM/IV) *and* diphenhydramine 1-2 mg/kg IV *and* methylprednisolone 2 mg/kg IV]. *Use epi with care in older patients or those with heart disease or HTN. If bronchospasm is present, administer bronchodilator therapy.*
Aortic dissection	[Propranolol 0.5 mg IV test dose—then after 5min start 1 mg IV Q5min until pulse 60-70 or 0.15 mg/kg given, then nitroprusside (dosing p. 155) to titrate BP to 100/60]; *or* labetalol 20 mg IV, then 40-80 mg IV Q 10min, titrate pulse/BP as above, max 300 mg; *or* labetalol start 2 mg/min infusion, titrate pulse/BP as above.
Arthritis, septic	
Child <3 month	[*Either* (methicillin* *or* nafcillin* *or* oxacillin*) *and either* (3rd gen ceph* *or* amikacin* *or* gentamicin* *or* tobramycin*)]. *Methicillin resistant staph. aureus:* vancomycin* . **Etiol:** *Staph. aureus, Enterobacteriaceae, Group B strep.*
Child 3 month-6 y.o.	[*Either* (methicillin* *or* nafcillin* *or* oxacillin* *or* 1st gen ceph*) *and* (3rd gen ceph*)]. Methicillin resistant *Staph. aureus:* vancomycin*. **Etiol:** *Staph. aureus, H. influenzae, Strep., Enterobacteriaceae.*

Adult, gonococcal	Use regimen for disseminated gonococcal infection p. 14.
Adult, non-gonococcal	[Either (methicillin* or nafcillin* or oxacillin* or 1st gen ceph*) and either (amikacin* or gentamicin* or tobramycin* or ciprofloxacin*)]; or ticarcillin/clav*; or ampicillin/sulbactam*; or piperacillin/tazobactam*. **Etiol:** *Staph. aureus, Group A strep., Enterobacteriaceae.*
Prosthetic joint, post-op, or post joint injection	[Vancomycin* and either (ciprofloxacin* or amikacin* or gentamicin* or tobramycin* or aztreonam*)]; or imipenem*. **Etiol:** *Staph. epidermidis, Staph. aureus, Enterobacteriaceae, Pseudomonas.*

Bites

Cat	Amoxicillin/clavulanate*; or PCN*; or ceftriaxone*; or doxycycline*. **Etiol:** *Pasteurella multocida, Staph. aureus.*
Dog	PCN*; or ampicillin*; or doxycycline*; or amoxicillin/clavulanate*; or ceftriaxone*. **Etiol:** *Viridans strep., Pasteurella multocida, Bacteroides, Fusobacterium.*
Human	Amoxicillin/clavulanate*; or PCN*; or ampicillin*; or erythromycin*; or cefoxitin*; or ampicillin/sulbactam*. **Etiol:** *Viridans strep., Staph. epidermidis, corynebacterium, Staph. aureus, Eikenella, Bacteroides, Peptostreptococcus.*
Pig (swine)	Amoxicillin/clavulanate*; or 3rd gen ceph*; or ticarcillin/clavulanate*; or ampicillin/sulbactam*; or imipenem*. **Etiol:** *Polymicrobial.*
Rat, bat, raccoon, skunk	Ampicillin*; or tetracycline*. **Etiol:** Rat: *Bacillus moniliformis.* Others: *unknown.*
Bursitis, septic	Dicloxacillin*; or cloxacillin*; or oxacillin*; or nafcillin*; or methicillin*; or 1st gen ceph* or vancomycin*; or [ciprofloxacin* (only if > 18 y.o.) and rifampin*]. **Etiol:** *Staph. aureus.*

Drug Therapy of Specific Disease Entities

For generic names of proprietary meds, see index

DISEASE	REGIMEN
Candida	
Oral (thrush) -no HIV	*Child 3 y.o.-adult:* Clotrimazole troches*; *or* nystatin susp*; *or* (adult only) fluconazole 100 mg po single dose.
Oral (thrush) or esophageal-with HIV	*Child:* Clotrimazole troches*; *or* nystatin susp*; *or 3-13 y.o.:* fluconazole 10 mg/kg po then 24h later start later start 3-6 mg/kg po QD.
	Child 13 y.o.-adult: Clotrimazole troches*; *or* nystatin susp*; *or* fluconazole 200 mg po, then 24h later start 100 mg po QD, up to 400 mg/d has been used.
	Treat AIDS patients for at least 3wk and for at least 2wk after resolution of symptoms.
Skin	Topical clotrimazole*; *or* miconazole*; *or* nystatin*.
Vaginitis	See *"vaginitis"*.
Cerebral edema	*Keep head of bed elevated as a general measure.*
Trauma, stroke, hepatic failure, Reye syndrome, glutethimide overdose (with signs of herniation)	
	Child/adult: Mannitol 0.25 g/kg IV ASAP, further doses of 0.25 mg/kg IV as needed, *and controlled hyperventilation to maintain pCO2 at 30 mm.*
Neoplasm, meningitis	*Child/adult:* Dexamethasone 0.15 mg/kg IV, then 0.08mg/kg IV Q 6h; if signs of herniation occur, add mannitol as above.
Chancroid	*Adult:* Azithromycin 1 g po single dose **preferred**; *or* ceftriaxone 250 mg IM single dose **preferred**; *or* erythromycin 500 mg po QID for 7d **preferred**; *or* amox/clav 500 mg (as amox) po TID for 7d; *or* ciprofloxacin 500 mg po BID for 3d.
Chlamydia infections	*Child <8 y.o, <45 kg:* Erythromycin 12.5 mg/kg/dose po QID for 10-14d.
	Child <8 y.o, >45 kg: Use adult erythromycin dosing given below for adults.

	Child >8 y.o.-adult: Doxycycline 100 mg po BID for 7d **preferred**; *or* azithromycin 1.0 g po single dose **preferred**; *or* ofloxacin 300 mg po BID for 7d *(only if > 18 y.o.);* *or* erythromycin base 500 mg po QID for 7d **preferred in pregnancy;** *or* erythromycin ethylsuccinate 800 mg po QID for 7d **preferred in pregnancy;** *or* sulfisoxazole 500 mg po QID for 10d *(inferior efficacy in comparison to others).*
Diabetic ketoacidosis	*Child/adult:* Regular insulin 0.1 U/kg IV, then infusion at 0.1 U/kg/h. Hydration with normal saline and appropriate monitoring are essential.
Diverticulitis	[Trimethoprim/sulfa* and metronidazole*]; *or* [ciprofloxacin* and metronidazole*]; *or* [*either* (amikacin* *or* gentamicin* *or* tobramycin*) *and either* (cefoxitin* *or* clindamycin*)]. **Etiol:** *Enterobacteriaceae, Bacteroides, Enterococci.*
Duodenal ulcer relapse *(Eradication of Helicobacter pylori)*	*Adult:* [PeptoBismol 525 mg po QID *and* metronidazole 250 mg po TID *and either* (amoxicillin 500 mg po QID *or* tetracycline 500 mg po QID)] for 14d; *or* [clarithromycin 500 mg po TID for 14d *and* omeprazole 40 mg QD for 14-28d].
Dysfunctional uterine bleeding	Medroxyprogesterone acetate *(Provera)* 10 mg po QD for 10d. Stress to patient that bleeding will stop, then after finishing progesterone will start again, perhaps heavily and with cramps, before abating.
Dystonic reaction, acute	*Adult:* Diphenhydramine 50 mg IM/IV, then 50 mg po QID for 3d; *or* benztropine mesylate *(Cogentin)* 1 mg IM/IV, then 1-2 mg po BID for 3d.
Eclampsia	Magnesium sulfate 4-6 g IV over 1h followed by 2 g/h infusion. *If BP >110 diast. after Mg:* Hydralazine 5 mg IV, then 5-10 mg IV Q20min as needed. *If seizures do not respond to Mg:* Diazepam 2-4 mg slow IV push.

* FOR DRUG DOSING SEE TABLE BEGINNING ON PAGE 36.

Drug Therapy of Specific Disease Entities   *For generic names of proprietary meds, see index*

DISEASE	REGIMEN

Endocarditis

Treatment – empiric therapy pending culture results:

Child/adult:

• Valvular or congenital heart disease or MVP

[(PCN G HD* *or* ampicillin* *or* vancomycin*) *and* gentamicin*]. *Omit gentamicin if pt >65 y.o. or has decreased hearing or renal function.*

Etiol: *Viridans strep, Strep bovis, Enterococci.*

• New onset CHF, new regurg. murmur, sepsis, pneumonia, meningitis

[(Nafcillin* *or* methicillin* *or* oxacillin *) *and* PCN G HD* *and* (amikacin* *or* gentamicin* *or* tobramycin*)].

Etiol: *Staph. aureus, Enterococci, S. pneumoniae, Group A strep.*

• IV drug use

Vancomycin* *and* gentamicin*.

Etiol: *Staph. aureus, Pseudomonas, Enterococci.*

Prophylaxis – American Heart Association recommendations, *JAMA* 1990; 264:2919.

Valvular conditions susceptible to endocarditis: any type prosthetic valve, previous bacterial endocarditis, most congenital cardiac defects, rheumatic or other acquired valve dysfunction, hypertrophic cardiomyopathy, mitral valve prolapse with valve regurgitation.

Procedures with risk: dental/surgical procedures causing mucosal or gingival bleeding (including teeth cleaning), tonsillectomy/adenoidectomy, procedure involvement of respiratory or intestinal mucosas, rigid bronchoscopy, sclerotherapy of esophageal varices, esophageal dilatation, gallbladder surgery, I and D of infected tissue, cystoscopy, urethral dilatation, prostatic surgery, urethral catheterization or urinary tract surgery if infection is present, vaginal hysterectomy or vaginal delivery when infection is present.

Higher risk patients: have a history of endocarditis or have an artificial heart valve in place.

Antibiotics and adult dosing:

Dental, oral, or upper respiratory tract procedures: amoxicillin 3.0 g po 1h before procedure, then 1.5 g po 6h later.

If PCN/amoxicillin allergic: erythromycin ethylsuccinate 800 mg (or eryth. stearate 1000 mg) po 2h before procedure, then ½ of initial dose 6h later; or clindamycin 300 mg po 1h before, then 150 mg 6h later.

If unable to take oral meds: ampicillin 2 g IM/IV 30min before procedure, then ampicillin 1 g IM/IV or amoxicillin 1.5 g po 6h later.

If unable to take oral meds and PCN allergic: clindamycin 300 mg IV 30min before procedure, then clindamycin 150 mg po/IV 6h later.

Higher risk patients: ampicillin 2 g and gentamicin 1.5 mg/kg (max 80 mg) IM/IV 30min before procedure, then amoxicillin 1.5 g po 6h later or repeat amp/gent IM/IV drug doses 8h after initial doses.

If higher risk and has PCN allergy: vancomycin 1 g IV over 1h starting 1h before procedure, single dose only.

Genitourinary or gastrointestinal procedures: ampicillin/gentamicin as for *higher risk* patients above.

If PCN/amoxicillin allergic: vancomycin 1 g IV over 1h starting 1h before procedure and gentamicin 1.5 mg/kg (max 80 mg) IM/IV 1h before procedure; repeat regimen 8h after initial doses.

Alternate low risk patient regimen: amoxicillin 3 g po 1h before procedure, then 1.5 g po 6h later.

Pediatric dosing (use same antibiotics and timing as for adults): amoxicillin or ampicillin 50 mg/kg; erythromycin ethylsuccinate or stearate 20 mg/kg; clindamycin 10 mg/kg; gentamicin 2 mg/kg; vancomycin 20 mg/kg. Total pediatric dose not to exceed adult dose. Second pediatric dose ½ of first dose.

---

* FOR DRUG DOSING SEE TABLE BEGINNING ON PAGE 36.

Drug Therapy of Specific Disease Entities

Disease	Regimen
Epididymo-orchitis	*Male <35 y.o.:* Treat for gonorrhea (p. 13), followed by treatment for chlamydia (p. 8). *Or:* Ofloxacin 300 mg po BID for 10d (*only if > 18 y.o.*). *Male >35 y.o.:* Trimethoprim/sulfa 1 double strength po BID for 14d; *or* ciprofloxacin*; *or* norfloxacin*; *or* ofloxacin*. *Severe disease:* Amoxicillin/clavulanate*; *or* ampicillin/sulbactam*; *or* 3rd gen ceph*; *or* ticarcillin/clavulanate*; *or* piperacillin/tazobactam*.
Epiglottitis	Cefuroxime*; *or* cefotaxime*; *or* ceftriaxone*; *or* ampicillin/sulbactam*; *or* trimeth/sulfa*. **Etiol:** Child-*H. influenzae;* Adult-*Group A strep, H. influenzae* (rare).
Gastroenteritis	
Infant e. coli culture positive Diarrhea with fever, bloody stool, tenesmus	Neomycin 25 mg/kg po Q6h; *or* colistin 3.75 mg/kg po Q6h. Ciprofloxacin* (*only if > 18 y.o.*); *or* trimeth/sulfa* for 3d. Loperamide* for diarrhea. *Culture for bacterial pathogens, send stool for O&P. If recently on antibiotics, consider C. difficile colitis, stop antibiotics if possible, send stool for C. difficile toxin, start cipro or trimeth/sulfa as above, add:*
Pseudomembranous colitis	*Child:* Metronidazole 5 mg/kg/dose po Q6h; *or* vancomycin 10-12.5 mg/kg/dose po Q6h (max 500 mg/d). *Adult:* Metronidazole 0.75-2 g/d po divided Q6-8h; *or* vancomycin 125 mg po Q6h. **Etiol:** *Shigella, Salmonella, Campylobacter jejuni, E. coli, C. difficile if recent antibiotics.*
Travel to tropics	Ciprofloxacin* (*only if > 18 y.o.*); *or* trimethoprim/sulfa*. Loperamide* for diarrhea. *Culture for bacterial pathogens, send stool for O&P.* **Etiol:** *tox. E. coli, Campylobacter jejuni, Salmonella, Shigella, Cyclospora cayetanesis.*

Recent seafood	Doxycycline*; or ciprofloxacin* *(only if > 18 y.o.)*. Fluid repletion indicated. *Culture for bact pathogens/send stool for O&P.* **Etiol:** *Vibrio cholera or parahemolyticus.*
Giardiasis	*Child:* Quinacrine 2 mg/kg/dose po TID after meals for 5d; *or* furazolidone 1.5 mg/kg/dose po QID for 10d *(only Rx available in liquid form)*; *or* metronidazole 5 mg/kg/dose po TID for 5d. *Do not exceed adult doses.* *Adult:* Metronidazole 250 mg po TID for 5d; *or* quinacrine 100 mg po TID after meals for 5d.
Glaucoma, acute angle closure	[Glycerol 50% 1 g (2 ml)/kg in chilled solution mixed with cold lemon juice *and* pilocarpine 2% 1 drop Q15min for 2-3h *and* timolol 0.5% 1 drop, repeat in 10min *and* acetazolamide 500 mg po *or* 250 mg IV. If cannot tolerate glycerol, consider mannitol 0.5-2.0 g/kg IV over 30-60min)].
Gonorrhea *Uncomplicated urethral, endocervical, or rectal infection*	*Treatment for chlamydia (p. 8) in addition to gonorrhea is mandatory.* *Child <45 kg:* Ceftriaxone 125 mg IM single dose. *If PCN-allergic:* spectinomycin 40 mg/kg (max 2 g) IM single dose. *Child >45 kg:* use adult treatment regimens except fluoroquinolones. *Adult:* Ceftriaxone 125 mg IM single dose **preferred;** *or* cefixime 400 mg po single dose **preferred;** *or* ciprofloxacin 500 mg po single dose *(only if > 18 y.o.)* **preferred;** *or* ofloxacin 400 mg po single dose *(only if > 18 y.o.)* **preferred;** *or* spectinomycin 2 g IM single dose; *or* cefotaxime 500 mg IM single dose; *or* ceftizoxime 500 mg IM single dose; *or* cefotetan 1 g IM single dose; *or* cefoxitin 2 g IM single dose.
Conjunctivitis	*Child >20 kg-adult:* Ceftriaxone 1 g IM single dose. Lavage infected eye once with saline. **gonorrhea** *continued*

* *For drug dosing see table beginning on page 36.*

Drug Therapy of Specific Disease Entities

For generic names of proprietary meds, see index

DISEASE	REGIMEN
Gonorrhea (continued)	
Disseminated *(Pustular skin rash,* *arthralgias, tenosynovitis* *septic arthritis)*	*Child <45 kg:* Ceftriaxone 50 mg/kg IM/IV QD for 7d. *Child > 45 kg-adult:* Start ceftriaxone 1 g IM/IV QD **preferred**; or ceftizoxime 1 g IV Q8h; or cefotaxime 1 g IV Q8h; or spectinomycin 2 g IM Q 12h. *Treat IM/IV until 24-48h after improvement occurs, then give either:* cefixime 400 mg po BID or ciprofloxacin 500 mg po BID (*only if >18 y.o.*) to complete total of 7d of therapy. See "epididymo-orchitis".
Epididymitis	*Adult:* Ceftriaxone 1-2 g IV Q12h. Rx *meningitis for 10-14d, endocard. for at least 3-4wk.*
Meningitis/endocarditis	
Ophthalmia neonatorum or infants born to mothers with untreated GC	*Newborn child:* Ceftriaxone 25-50 mg/kg (max 125 mg) single dose IM/IV.
Pharyngitis	*Adult:* Ceftriaxone 250 mg IM single dose; or ciprofloxacin 500 mg po single dose.
Gout, acute attack	*Adult:* Indomethacin 75 mg po, then 50 mg po Q 6h until 24h after relief, then 50 mg po Q 8h for 3 doses, then 25 mg po Q 8h for 3 doses; or Colchicine 0.5-0.6 mg po Q 1h or 1.0 mg po Q 2h until either relief, occurence of GI sx, or when 6 mg has been given without relief; or Colchicine 2-3 mg IV, then 1 mg IV Q 6h (max total 4 mg) until relief is obtained. Dilute with 20 ml NS. *Fewer GI problems than with po administration.*
Headache, migraine	*Adult:* [Ketorolac 30-60 mg IM *and* sumatriptan 6 mg SC]; or [Metoclopramide 10 mg IV, then dihydroergotamine 0.75-1.0 mg IV]. *To either regimen may add:* [Either (meperidine 75-150 mg IM *or* hydromorphone 1-3 mg IM) *with or without* hydroxyzine 50 mg IM].

Hemophilia	See p. 168.
Hepatitis B exposure	*Child/adult:* Hepatitis B immune globulin (HBIG) 0.06 ml/kg IM in deltoid muscle as early as possible within 14d *and* Hepatitis B vaccine (for dosing see p. 67).
Herpes simplex	
Primary genital	Acyclovir 200 mg po 5 times/day *or* 400 mg po TID. Treat for 10d or until clinical resolution occurs.
Primary rectal	Acyclovir 400 mg po 5 times/day. Treat for 10d or until clinical resolution occurs.
Severe disease requiring hospitalization	Acyclovir 5-10 mg/kg IV Q 8h for 5-7d or until clinical resolution; *or if HIV+ and disease resistant to acyclovir:* foscarnet 40 mg/kg IV Q 8h until lesions heal (10-24d).
Encephalitis	Acyclovir 12.4 mg/kg IV Q 8h for 10d or longer.
Mucocutaneous (immunocompromised host)	Acyclovir 5 mg/kg IV Q 8h; *or* 200 mg po 5 times/day. Treat for 7d.
Recurrent genital	Acyclovir 200 mg po 5 times/day; *or* 400 mg po TID; *or* 800 mg po BID. Treat for 5d.
Daily suppressive	Acyclovir 400 mg po BID; *or* 200 mg po 3-5 times/day.
Keratitis	Trifluridine 1% one drop Q 2h (max 8 drops/d) for maximum 21d.
Hypertensive crisis	Nitroprusside start at 0.5 µg/kg/min, titrate to dose which controls BP (see p. 155 for dosing chart); *or*
	Labetalol 20 mg IV, then 40-80 mg IV Q 10min, max total 300 mg; *or*
	Labetalol start 2 mg/min infusion, titrate to desired BP.

* *FOR DRUG DOSING SEE TABLE BEGINNING ON PAGE 36.*

Drug Therapy of Specific Disease Entities

For generic names of proprietary meds, see index

DISEASE	REGIMEN
Hyperthyroidism (*Thyroid storm*)	*Adult:* [(Propranolol 1 mg/Q 5min IV to achieve sinus rate <100 BPM, max 10 mg, or if less severe disease 40-100 mg po Q 6h) *and* (propylthiouracil (PTU) 800-1200 mg po initially, then 300 mg po Q 6h) *and* beginning 2h after PTU *either* (Na iodide 125 mg/h by continuous infusion *or* Lugol's iodine 10 drops po Q 8h) *and* (hydrocortisone 100 mg IV)]. *Use acetaminophen, not aspirin, for fever. Send TSH, T3, T4. Supportive therapy essential, and may include digitalis for arrhythmias.*
Hypothyroid coma (*Myxedema coma*)	*Adult:* L-thyroxine 400 μg IV over 5min, *and* hydrocortisone 100 mg IV, then L-thyroxine 25 μg IV Q 6h. *Send TSH, T3, T4. Supportive therapy essential.*
Lice	*After treating lice, decontaminate clothing and bedding with washing machine on hot cycle or with dry cleaning. Treat household, close, and sexual contacts.*
Body Head Pubic	Pyrethrins with piperonyl butoxide (RID) apply and wash off in 10min. Wash hair, apply permethrin 1% liquid lotion for 10min. Rinse off and comb hair. Lindane 1% shampoo apply for 4min, then wash off thoroughly *(do not use if preg. or <2 y.o.); or* permethrin 1% creme rinse apply and wash off in 10min; *or* pyrethrins with piperonyl butoxide (RID) apply and wash off in 10min.
Lyme disease Tick bite	Antibiotic Rx not indicated for most tick bites. Transmission occurs in 10% of bites by infected ticks. To be cost-effective, risk of transmission needs to be ≥1%
Early (*erythema chronicum migrans*),	*Child* <9 y.o.: Amoxicillin 8.3-17 mg/kg/dose (max 1-2 g/d) po TID **preferred;** *or* if PCN-allergic, cefuroxime axetil 20 mg/kg/dose po BID; *or* erythromycin

or isolated facial palsy, or mild carditis	7.5 mg/kg/dose (max 1 g/d) po QID. *All for 10-28d, depending on response.* *Child 9 y.o.-adult:* Doxycycline 100 mg po BID for 10-21d **preferred**; *or* amoxicillin 500 mg po TID for 10-21d **preferred**; *or* cefuroxime axetil 500 mg po BID for 21d; *or* azithromycin 500 mg po, then 250 mg po QD for 4 more days; *or* clarithromycin 500 mg po BID for 21d.
Arthritis	*Child (initial treatment):* Use oral regimens. *Child (persistent arthritis):* Ceftriaxone 75-100 mg/kg (max 2 g) IM/IV QD for 14-30d. *Adult:* Doxycycline 100 mg po BID for 30d; *or* ceftriaxone 2 g IM/IV QD for 14d.
Severe carditis	*Child:* Ceftriaxone 75-100 mg/kg/d (max 2 g/dose) IM/IV QD; *or* PCN 50,000 U/kg/dose (max 20 million U/d) IV Q4h for 14-30d. *Adult:* Ceftriaxone 2 g IV QD for 14d; *or* cefotaxime* for 14d; *or* PCN HD* for 14d.
Meningitis	*Child:* Ceftriaxone 75-100 mg/kg/d (max 2 g/dose) IV QD; *or* PCN 50,000 U/kg/dose (max 20 million U/d) IV Q4h for 14-30d. *Adult:* Ceftriaxone 2 g IV QD for 21d; *or* PCN HD* for 21d.
Lymphogranuloma	*Adult:* Doxycycline 100 mg po BID for 21d **preferred**; *or* erythromycin 500 mg po QID for 21d; *or* sulfisoxazole 500 mg po QID for 21d.
Mastitis	
Postpartum	1st gen ceph*; *or* dicloxacillin*; *or* cloxacillin*; *or* oxacillin*; *or* nafcillin*; *or* methicillin*; *or* vancomycin*. **Etiol:** *Staph. aureus.*
Other	Clindamycin*; *or* [metronidazole* *and either* (1st gen ceph* *or* oxacillin* *or* dicloxacillin* *or* nafcillin* *or* methicillin*)]; *or* [vancomycin *and* metronidazole]. **Etiol:** *Staph. aureus, Bacteroides, Peptococcus.*

* FOR DRUG DOSING SEE TABLE BEGINNING ON PAGE 36.

Drug Therapy of Specific Disease Entities

DISEASE	REGIMEN
Meningitis *Treatment*	*For all children or adults with signs of increased ICP or significant CNS dysfunction: 15-20min before giving antibiotics start dexamethasone 0.15 mg/kg IV Q 6h IV for 4d (NEJM 324:1512) or 0.4 mg/kg IV Q 12h for 2d (Lancet 324:457) to improve outcome.*
Infant <1 month	[Ampicillin* and gentamicin* and 3rd gen ceph*]. **Etiol:** Group B or D strep, Enterobacteriaceae, Listeria.
Infant 1-3 month	[Ampicillin* and either (cefotaxime* or ceftriaxone*)]; or [chloramphenicol* and gentamicin*]. **Etiol:** H. influenzae, Pneumococci, Meningococci, and same as infant <1 mo. old.
Child 3 month-7 y.o.	Ceftriaxone*; or cefotaxime*; or ampicillin*. **Etiol:** H. influenzae (much less common if immunized), Pneumococci, Meningococci.
Child 7 y.o.-adult 50 y.o.	[(Ceftriaxone* or cefotaxime*) and (PCN G HD* or ampicillin*)]. *PCN-allergy mild:* ceftriaxone* or cefotaxime*. *PCN-allergy severe:* [chloramphenicol* and trimethoprim/sulfa*]. *Community with more than 2% S. pneumoniae PCN-resistant:* vancomycin IV* and 3rd gen ceph IV* and rifampin* and consider vancomycin inthrathecal. **Etiol:** Pneumococci, Meningococci, Listeria monocytogenes.
Adult >50 y.o. or medically complicated	[Vancomycin IV* and 3rd gen ceph IV* and rifampin IV* with or without vancomycin intrathecal]; or [chloramphenicol* and trimethoprim/sulfa*]. **Etiol:** Pneumococci most common, Enterobacteriaceae, H. flu, Listeria, Pseudomonas.
HIV infection	**Etiol:** Cryptococcus most common, also consider TB, syphilis, aseptic HIV infection, Listeria monocytogenes, and organisms seen in those >50 y.o.

For cryptococcus: amphotericin 0.5-0.8 mg/kg/d IV, until afebrile and resolution of N,V, headache, *then* fluconazole 400 mg po QD to complete 8-10wk course, *then* fluconazole 100-200 mg/d po as suppressive measure indefinitely.

	Vancomycin* and ceftazidime*. *For Pseudomonas add:* gentamicin IV/ intrathecal*.
	Etio: Staph. aureus, Enterobacteriaceae, Pseudomonas, Pneumococci.
Post neurosurg. procedure or craniospinal trauma Persistent CNS leak	Cefotaxime* or ceftriaxone*. **Etio: Pneumococci.**
V-P or other CNS shunt	Vancomycin* and rifampin*. *If g neg's on g-stain, add:* 3rd gen ceph. **Etio: Staph. epidermidis, Diphtheroids, Enterobacteriaceae.**

Prophylaxis

H. influenzae meningitis: *Child/adult:* rifampin 20 mg/kg (max 600 mg) po QD for 4d. *Indications:* 1) all household contacts regardless of age in households with any incompletely vaccinated contact <48 mo. old. *Household contact* = living with index pt (IP), or spent ≥4hr with IP for 5 of 7d before dx of IP, 2) *single case* at child care locale/nursery school: if attended by unvaccinated or incompletely vaccinated child <2 y.o. and children contact each other ≥25h/wk, treat all attendees, vaccinated or not. *If ≥2 cases:* treat all attendees and supervisory personnel, regardless of contact hours.

Meningococcal meningitis: *Child/adult:* rifampin 10 mg/kg/dose *(adult dose and max child dose 600 mg)* po BID for 2d *generally preferred; or* ceftriaxone 125 mg *(child <12 y.o.)* or 250 mg *(child 12 y.o.-adult)* IM **preferred if preg;** *or* sulfisoxazole 500 mg QD *(child <1 y.o.)* or 500 mg BID *(child 1-12 y.o.)* or 1 g BID *(child 12 y.o.-adult)* po for 2d **preferred if strain known sulfa sensitive;** *or* ciprofloxacin 500 mg single dose *(only if ≥18 y.o.)*. *Indications:* 1) *all* household, child care, nursery school contacts; 2) contact with oral secretions through kissing or sharing food/drink; 3) **not** medical personnel, unless intimate contact such as intubation, suctioning, etc. Treat ASAP, preferably within 24h.

* FOR DRUG DOSING SEE TABLE BEGINNING ON PAGE 36.

Drug Therapy of Specific Disease Entities

For generic names of proprietary meds, see index

DISEASE	REGIMEN

Myasthenia gravis

Diagnosis
"Tension test"

If cholinergic reaction occurs during tensilon test or emergency treatment, be prepared to give atropine 0.01-0.04 mg/kg (child) or 0.5 mg (adult).

Child >1 month: Edrophonium 1 mg (<34 kg) or 2 mg (>34 kg) IV over 15sec. If no response in 45sec, give 1 mg Q 30sec, max 5 mg (<34 kg) or 10 mg (>34 kg) IV.

Adult: Obtain edrophonium 10 mg in syringe. Give 2 mg IV over 15-30sec. If no response in 45sec, give remaining 8 mg IV over 30sec.

Positive test = objective improvement in contractility as well as subjective response.

Emergency treatment

Child: Neostigmine 0.01-0.04 mg/kg/dose SC/IM/IV Q 2-3h prn.
Adult: Neostigmine 0.5-2.5 mg SC/IM/IV Q4h.

Myocardial infarction

Thrombolytics

Accelerated ("front-loaded") t-PA (tissue plasminogen activator): 15 mg IVP, then 0.75 mg/kg (max 50 mg) over 30min, then 0.5 mg/kg (max 35 mg) over 1h; or

Regular t-PA regimen: 10 mg IVP, then 50 mg over 1h, then 20 mg/h for 2h; or

Streptokinase: 1.5 million U IV over 1h.

NEJM '93; 329:673 (GUSTO)—accel. t-PA reduced mortality compared with other 'lytic regimens.

Absolute contraindications: active internal bleeding, stroke last 3 mo., recent head trauma, known brain neoplasm, poss. aortic dissection, pregnancy, likely to have cardiac cath./angioplasty acutely, onset of sx longer than 6h ago in absence of ongoing ischemia. *Known hypersensitivity to streptokinase or previous use of streptokinase contraindicates its use.*

Relative contraindications: age ≥70 y.o., hx of CVA, recent vigorous CPR, internal jugular or subclavian or arterial puncture, major surgery/trauma last 6wk, hx severe uncontrolled HTN, significant liver dysfunction, stool positive for occult blood (may represent ASA effect).

Adjunctive	Aspirin 325 mg po at the time of presentation.
	Heparin 110 U/kg IV loading dose with start of thrombolytic infusion, then 15 U/kg/h.
	Beta-blockade: Metoprolol 5 mg IVP Q 5min × 3 (total 15 mg), then 15min later start 50 mg po Q6h for 48h, then 100 mg po Q12h for at least 3mo. If entire IV loading dose not tolerated, may reduce subsequent po dosing to 100 mg/d. *Other β-blockers shown to be effective. Best effect if administered within 4h of onset of symptoms.*
	Halt or do not start β-blocker for any of the following: hx bronchial asthma, 2nd or 3rd degree heart block or P-R >.24sec, rales >¹/₃ up lung fields or wheezing on exam, HR <50 BPM, systolic BP >95; PAP wedge >20-24.

Osteomyelitis

Newborn	[(Nafcillin* *or* methicillin*) *and* 3rd gen ceph*].
	Etiol: *Staph. aureus, Enterobacteriaceae, Group A and B strep.*
Child <4 years	3rd gen ceph*; *or* cefuroxime*.
	Etiol: *H. influenzae, Streptococci, Staph. aureus.*
Child >4 years	Nafcillin*; *or* methicillin*; *or* oxacillin*; *or* 1st gen ceph*; *or* vancomycin*; *or* clindamycin*.
	Etiol: *Staph. aureus, Streptococci, H. influenzae.*
Adult	Nafcillin*; *or* methicillin*; *or* oxacillin*; *or* 1st gen ceph*; *or* [ciprofloxacin* *and* rifampin*]; *or* [vancomycin* *and* 3rd gen. ceph*].
	Etiol: *Staph. aureus*—*Enterobacteriaceae and Streptococci much less common.*
Post-op or post trauma	[Ciprofloxacin* *(only if* >18 y.o.) *and* rifampin*]; *or* ticarcillin/clavulanate*; *or* [vancomycin* *and* 3rd gen ceph*]; *or* imipenem*.
	Etiol: *Staph. aureus, Enterobacteriaceae, Pseudomonas.* **osteomyelitis** *continued*

* *FOR DRUG DOSING SEE TABLE BEGINNING ON PAGE 36.*

Drug Therapy of Specific Disease Entities

DISEASE	REGIMEN
Osteomyelitis (continued)	
Nail puncture of foot	Ciprofloxacin* *(only if > 18 y.o.); or* ticarcillin/clav*; *or* imipenem*; *or* cefoperazone*; *or* ceftazidime*. **Etiol:** *Pseudomonas, Staph. aureus is much less common.*
Vertebral	*Post laminectomy:* Nafcillin*; *or* methicillin*; *or* oxacillin*; *or* vancomycin*. **Etiol:** *Staph. aureus, Staph. epidermidis.*
	Blood-borne: [Ciprofloxacin* *(only if > 18 y.o.) and* rifampin*]; *or* ticarcillin/clav*; *or* [vancomycin* *and* 3rd gen ceph*]; *or* imipenem*. **Etiol:** *Staph. aureus, Enterobacteriaceae, P. aeruginosa, candida.*
Pelvic inflammatory disease	
Inpatient	*Admit if:* dx unclear, possible surgical emergency, possible pelvic abscess, pregnant, adolescent pt, severe illness, patient cannot tolerate outpatient therapy, outpatient therapy has failed, patient cannot follow-up in 72h, patient is HIV+.
	[(Cefoxitin 2 g IV Q 6h *or* cefotetan 2 g IV Q 12h) *and* doxycycline 100 mg po or IV Q 12h]; *or*
	Gentamicin loading 2 mg/kg IM/IV, then gentamicin 1.5 mg/kg IM/IV Q 8h, *and* clindamycin 900 mg IV Q 8h.
	Continue IV antibiotics for 48h after substantial clinical improvement, then start and continue to complete 14d of therapy: doxycycline 100 mg po BID; *or for clindamycin regimen either:* doxycycline 100 mg po BID *or* clindamycin 450 mg po QID.
Outpatient	[(Cefoxitin 2 g IM with probenecid 1 g po *or* ceftriaxone 250 mg IM), then doxycycline 100 mg po BID for 14d].

Peritonitis

Spontaneous bacterial

[Ampicillin* and either (amikacin* or gentamicin* or tobramycin*)]; or cefoxitin*; or ampicillin/sulbactam*; or ticarcillin/clavulanate*; or piperacillin/tazobactam.
Etiol: *Enterobacteriaceae, Staph. aureus, S. pneumoniae, Group A strep.*

Bowel perforation

[Ampicillin* and metronidazole* and either (amikacin* or gentamicin* or tobramycin*)]; or cefoxitin*; or cefotetan*; or ampicillin/sulbactam*; or ticarcillin/clavulanate*; or imipenem*.
Etiol: *Enterobacteriaceae, enterococci, Bacteroides, Pseudomonas aeruginosa.*

Pertussis

Child/adult: Erythromycin 12.5 mg/kg/dose (max and adult dose 2 g/d) po QID for 14d **preferred;** or trimethoprim/sulfa (as trimeth) 4 mg/kg/dose po BID for 14d. *Child may re-enter day care 5 days after start of treatment.*
Unimmunized close contacts: initiate DTP, give erythromycin 12.5 mg/kg/dose *(child)* or 500 mg po QID *(adult)* for 14d. *Observe day care contacts for 14d.*

Pharyngitis

Diphtheric (membranous)

Child/adult: Erythromycin 10-12.5 mg/kg/dose (max and adult dose 2 g/d) po/IV Q6h for 14d; or aqueous PCN G 100,000-150,00 U/kg/d IM divided Q6h for 14d; or procaine PCN G 25,000-50,000 U/kg/d IM divided Q12h for 14d.
Equine antitoxin should be given as soon as possible.
Close contacts: 1) Observe closely for 7d; 2) culture for diphtheria; 3) prophylax with either erythromycin 10-12.5 mg/kg/dose (max and adult dose 2 g/d) Q6h for 7d; or benzathine PCN G 600,000 U *(<30 kg)* or 1.2 million U *(>30 kg)* IM single dose. See p. 14.

Gonococcal

pharyngitis *continued*

Drug Therapy of Specific Disease Entities

For generic names of proprietary meds, see index

DISEASE	REGIMEN
Pharyngitis (continued) *Streptococcal*	*Child/adult:* Benzathine PCN 600,000 U (<27 kg) or 1.2 MU (>27 kg) IM; or PCN VK 250 mg po TID for 10d. *If PCN allergic:* erythromycin estolate 20-40 mg/kg/d (max & adult dose 1 g/d) po divided BID or QID for 10d; or erythro ethyl succinate 40-50 mg/kg/d (max & adult dose 1 g/d) po div TID-QID for 10d.
Pneumocystis pneumonia *New onset pneumonia– clinical AIDS or HIV+ with CD4 <200/mm³*	Start suppressive therapy after completing course. *Child:* Trimethoprim/sulfa (as trimeth) 15-20 mg/kg/d po/IV divided Q 6-8h for 14-21d **preferred;** or pentamidine 3-4 mg/kg IV QD for 14-21d. *If >13 y.o. and pO₂ <70,* add prednisone 40 mg po BID for 5d, then 20 mg po QD for 11d with first dose prior to initial anti-pneumocystis therapy. Although most feel younger hypoxic children would benefit from steroids, optimal dose and course not established. *Adult:* **Mild disease (not acutely ill, pO₂ >70, can take oral meds):** Trimeth/sulfa 2 DS tabs (as trimeth = 3.75-5 mg/kg/dose) po QID for 21d **preferred;** or [trimethoprim 5 mg/kg/dose po Q6h *and* dapsone 100 mg po QD for 21d]; or or [primaquine base 30 mg po QD *and* clindamycin 900 mg po/IV Q6h for 21d]; or atovaquone 750 mg po TID for 21d. **Severe disease (acutely ill, pO₂ <70, cannot take oral meds):** Trimethoprim/sulfa (as trimeth) 20 mg/kg/d IV divided Q 6-8h for 21d **preferred;** or pentamidine 4 mg/kg IV QD for 21d; or pentamidine 600 mg in 6 ml sterile water by nebulizer QD for 21d; or [trimetrexate 45 mg/m² IV QD for 21d *and* folinic acid 20 mg po/IV q 6h for 24d]. *Start prednisone 40 mg po BID for 5d, then 20 mg po QD for 11d with first dose PT initial anti-pneumocystis Rx.*

Prophylaxis	*Child:* Trimethoprim/sulfa (as trimeth) 75 mg/m² (max 80 mg/dose) po BID given every day or 3 times/wk **preferred**; *or* dapsone 1 mg/kg/dose po QD; *or* (only if >5 y.o.) pentamidine 4 mg/kg/dose IM Q 2 wk-1 mo. *Adult:* Trimeth/sulfa 1 DS tab po 3 times/wk **preferred**; *or* dapsone 50-100 mg po QD; *or* pentamidine 300 mg in 6 ml sterile water Q month by special aerosol device.

Pneumonia

Child <5d old at onset	[Ampicillin* *and* gentamicin*]; *or* 3rd gen ceph*. **Etiol:** *E. coli; Group A, B, G strep.*
Child ≥5d-1 month old	[*Either* (methicillin* *or* nafcillin* *or* oxacillin*) *and* gentamicin*]. *Methicillin resistant staph. aureus:* vancomycin*. **Etiol:** *Group A or B or G strep., Staph. aureus, E. coli, Pseudomonas, chlamydia.*
Child 1 month-5 y.o.	Ceftriaxone*; *or* cefotaxime*; *or* [*either* (nafcillin* *or* methicillin* *or* oxacillin*) *and either* (amikacin* *or* gentamicin* *or* tobramycin*)]. **Etiol:** *viral, Strep. pneumoniae, H. influenzae, Staph. aureus.*
Child 5 y.o.-adult 40 y.o. w/o underlying disease	
G stain: non-diagnostic	Azithromycin* *or* clarithromycin* *or* erythromycin*. *Based on severity, either:* PCN LD* *or* PCN VK 500 mg po QID. *PCN-allergy:* erythromycin*; *or* trimethoprim/sulfa*; *or* azithromycin*; *or* clarithromycin*; *or* clindamycin*; *or* chloramphenicol*; *or* vancomycin*. *Community with 2% PCN-resist. pneumococcus:* start vancomycin* , *then, depending on suscept. testing:* cefotaxime*; *or* ceftriaxone*; *or* chloramphenicol*; *or* PCN HD* .
G stain: pneumococci	
G stain: H. influenzae	Ampicillin/sulbactam*; *or* amox/clav*; *or* 2nd or 3rd gen ceph*. **Etiol:** *mycoplasma, chlamydia, Strep. pneumoniae, Legionella, H. influenzae.* **pneumonia** *continued*

* *For drug dosing see table beginning on page 36.*

Drug Therapy of Specific Disease Entities

DISEASE	REGIMEN
Pneumonia (continued)	
>40 y.o. with no underlying disease	Ceftriaxone*; or cefotaxime*; or cefuroxime*; or trimethoprim/sulfa*; or amoxicillin/clavulanate; or ampicillin/sulbactam*; or ticarcillin/clavulanate*; or azithromycin*; or clarithromycin*. *Community with 2% PCN-resist. pneumococcus: treat patient as for PCN-resistant pneumococcus above.* **Etiol:** *Strep. pneumoniae, Group A strep., H. influenzae, mycoplasma.*
>40 y.o. with alcoholism, diabetes, CHF, other underlying disease	[Erythromycin* and either (ceftriaxone* or cefotaxime* or amoxicillin/clavulanate* or ampicillin/sulbactam* or ticarcillin/clavulanate*; or imipenem*)]
Aspiration	**Etiol:** *as for healthy >40 y.o., also: gram neg's, Legionella, chlamydia, Staph. aureus.* [Clindamycin* and gentamicin*]; or cefoxitin*; or ampicillin/sulbactam*; or ticarcillin/clavulanate*; or piperacillin/tazobactam*. **Etiol:** *Strep. pneumoniae, Bacteroides, other oral flora.*
IV drug use	[Either (amikacin* or gentamicin* or tobramycin)* and either (methicillin* or nafcillin* or vancomycin*)]. **Etiol:** *Staph. aureus, gram negatives (less common).*
Neutropenia (PMN <500/mm³)	Imipenem*; or [either (amikacin* or gentamicin* or tobramycin*) and either (carbenicillin* or ticarcillin* or piperacillin* or mezlocillin or ceftazidime* or ceftazidime* or cefoperazone*) with or without vancomycin*]. **Etiol:** *gram negatives, Staph. aureus, Legionella, candida, aspergillus, Mucor-Rhizopus.*
Pneumocystis	See *"pneumocystis".*

Prostatitis, acute

Male <35 y.o.   Treat for GC (p. 13), followed by treatment for chlamydia (p. 8).
Etiol: *GC, chlamydia.*

Male >35 y.o.   Ciprofloxacin*; *or* norfloxacin*; *or* ofloxacin*; *or* trimethoprim/sulfa*.
Etiol: *Enterobacteriaceae.*

Pulmonary embolus

Treatment   *Child:* Heparin 50 U/kg IV, then infusion at 10-25 U/kg/h.
Adult: Heparin 70-100 units/kg IV, then infusion at 15 U/kg/h.
Consider thrombolytics for massive PE with hemodynamic compromise. Dosing on p. 34.

Prophylaxis   *Pre-op or bed-ridden:* Heparin 70-125 U/kg SC Q12h.

Rabies prophylaxis   *Child/adult:* [Local wound cleansing with soap and water] *and* [rabies immune globulin* (RIG) 20 IU/kg, ½ of dose infiltrated around wound(s) if possible, remainder IM in gluteal area] *and* [rabies vaccine* HDCV or RVA 1.0 ml IM in deltoid (younger children outer aspect of thigh) on days 0, 3, 7, 14, 28].
See p. 140 for indications for giving RIG and vaccine.

Rape   Ceftriaxone 125 mg IM single dose *and* doxycycline 100 mg po BID for 7d. Hepatitis B prophylaxis with Hepatitis B immune globulin (HBIG) 0.06 ml/kg IM in deltoid muscle *and* Hepatitis B vaccine (for dosing see p. 67) suggested. Culture for gonorrhea/chlamydia, do wet mount for trichomonas, save serum for analysis if follow-up serology positive. Follow-up at 2wk and 12wk after assault. Check syphilis/HIV serologies at 12wk visit. Evidence collection and psych/social support essential. *Based on CDC recommendations from MMWR 1993; 42, #RR-14.*

---

* *FOR DRUG DOSING SEE TABLE BEGINNING ON PAGE 36.*

Drug Therapy of Specific Disease Entities

DISEASE	REGIMEN
Scabies	*Child/adult:* Permethrin 5% cream 60 g. Apply from neck down, wash off in 8-14h. **Preferred;** *or*
	Lindane 1% cream (30 g) or lotion (1 oz). Apply thinly from neck down, wash off in 8h. **Preferred** *but do not use if pregnant or breast feeding, for child <2 y.o., or if extensive dermatitis is present; or*
	Crotamiton 10%. Apply from neck down nightly for 2 consecutive nights, wash off 24h after last application.
	Wash clothing and bedsheets or remove these from body contact for 72h. Re-examine in 7d. May need to re-treat. Examine and treat close personal contacts.
Sepsis, unknown source	
Child ≤4d old	[Ampicillin* *and either* (cefotaxime* *or* amikacin* *or* gentamicin* *or* tobramycin*)].
	Etiol: *Group B strep., E. coli, klebsiella, enterobacter, Staph. aureus.*
Child 5d-1 month old	[Ampicillin* *and either* (cefotaxime* *or* ceftriaxone* *or* amikacin* *or* gentamicin* *or* tobramycin*)].
	Etiol: *Group B strep., E. coli, klebsiella, enterobacter, Staph. aureus, H. influenzae.*
Child >1 month old, not immunocompromised	Cefotaxime*, *or* ceftriaxone*; *or* cefuroxime*; *or* amp/sulbactam* *or* amox/clav* .
	Etiol: *H. influenzae, Strep. pneumoniae, meningococci, Staph. aureus.*
Adult, not immunocompromised	[*Either* (3rd gen ceph* *or* carbenicillin* *or* ticarcillin* *or* piperacillin* *or* mezlocillin* *or* ticarcillin/clavulanate* *or* piperacillin/tazobactam* *or* cefoxitin*) *and either* (amikacin* *or* gentamicin* *or* tobramycin*)]; *or* [ampicillin* *and* clindamycin* *and either* (amikacin* *or* gentamicin* *or* tobramycin*)]; *or* imipenem* .
	Etiol: *Gram positive cocci, Gram negative aerobic bacilli, anaerobes.*

Neutropenia (PMN <500/mm³)	*Child/adult: [Either* (carbenicillin* *or* ticarcillin* *or* piperacillin* *or* mezlocillin* *or* ceftazidime* *or* cefoperazone*) *and either* (amikacin* *or* gentamicin* *or* tobramycin*) plus vancomycin* *if catheter implicated]; or* imipenem*. **Etiol:** *Enterobacteriaceae, Pseudomonas, Staph. aureus or epidermidis, Viridans strep.*
Splenectomized	*Child/adult:* Cefotaxime*; *or* ceftriaxone*. **Etiol:** *Strep. pneumoniae, H. influenzae, meningococci.*
IV drug use	*Adult: [Either* (methicillin* *or* nafcillin* *or* oxacillin* *or* vancomycin*) *and either* (amikacin* *or* gentamicin* *or* tobramycin*)]. **Etiol:** *Staph. aureus, gram negative bacilli less common.*
Sinusitis *Acute*	*Topical nasal and oral decongestants should also be prescribed.* *Child/adult:* Trimethoprim/sulfa*; *or* amoxicillin/clavulanate*; *or oral 2nd or 3rd gen ceph*; or* clarithromycin*. **Etiol:** *Strep pneumoniae, H. influenzae, M. catarrhalis, Group A strep., anaerobes, viruses, Staph. aureus.*
Chronic	*Child:* Erythromycin/sulfa* *(Pediazole); or* amoxicillin/clavulanate*; *or oral 2nd or 3rd gen ceph*. **Etiol:** *Strep. pneumoniae, H. influenzae, M. catarrhalis. Adult: antibiotics usually ineffective unless sx acute—ENT consult usually indicated.* **Etiol:** *Bacteroides, Peptostreptococci, Fusobacterium.*
Spinal cord injury, acute	*Acute trauma, new cord deficit:* methylprednisolone 30 mg/kg IV over 15min, then 45min later start infusion at 5.4 mg/kg/h for 23h.

* *FOR DRUG DOSING SEE TABLE BEGINNING ON PAGE 36.*

Drug Therapy of Specific Disease Entities

For generic names of proprietary meds, see index

DISEASE	REGIMEN

Syphilis

<1 yr duration (primary or secondary)

Child: Benzathine PCN G 50,000 U/kg (max 2.4 million U) single dose IM.
Adult: Benzathine PCN G 2.4 MU IM **preferred**; *or* doxycycline 100 mg po BID for 14d; *or* tetracycline 500 mg po QID for 14d.

>1 yr duration (late latent, cardiovascular, late benign)

Child: Benzathine PCN G 50,000 U/kg (max 2.4 MU) IM Q wk for 3 doses.
Adult: Benthazine PCN 2.4 million U IM Q wk for 3 doses **preferred**; *or* doxycycline 100 mg po BID for 4wk; *or* tetracycline 500 mg po QID for 4wk.

Neurosyphilis

PCN G 2-4 million U IV Q 4h for 10-14d **preferred**; *or* [procaine PCN 2.4 million U IM QD *and* probenecid 500 mg po QID for 10-14d].
After either neurosyphilis regimen: Benthazine PCN 2.4 million U IM Q wk for 3 doses.

Tinea

†*Griseofulvin doses here are given for "microsize" preparation—see p. 66.*

Capitis

Child >2 y.o.: Griseofulvin† 10-20 mg/kg/dose (max 1000 mg/d) po QD for 4-6wk; *or* ketoconazole 3.3-6.6 mg/kg/dose po QD for 4wk.
Adult: Griseofulvin† 0.5-1 g po QD for 4-6wk; *or* ketoconazole 200 mg po QD for 4wk.

Corporis

Child/adult: Topical miconazole* or clotrimazole* BID for 2-4wk. If one of these is unsuccessful, consider ketoconazole 200 mg po QD for at least 4wk for adults or griseofulvin* for children.

Cruris or pedis

Child/adult: Topical miconazole* or clotrimazole* BID for 2-4 weeks.

Unguium (onychomycosis)

Child/adult: Griseofulvin† 10-20 mg/kg/d (max 1000 mg/d) po divided BID or QD. for 3-4 months (*fingernails*) or 6 months (*toenails*).

Versicolor

Child: Topical ketoconazole* for 2wk; *or* 2.5% selenium sulfide lotion* QD for 7d.
Adult: Ketoconazole 400 mg po as a single dose.

Toxoplasmosis
Treatment

Without AIDS: *Child:* [Pyrimethamine 1 mg/kg/dose po BID for 1-3d, then 1 mg/kg po QD *and* sulfadiazine 100 mg/kg/d (max 8 g/d) divided TID-QID *and* folinic acid 5-10 mg po QD]. *Treat for 4-5 weeks.*
Adult: [Pyrimethamine 100 mg po on day 1, then 25 mg po QD *and* sulfadiazine 4-6 g/d po QD *and* folinic acid 10 mg po QD]. *Treat for 4-5 weeks.*
With AIDS: *Child:* same regimen as without AIDS. *Treat for 4-5 weeks.*
Adult: [Pyrimethamine 100 mg po BID, then 50-75 mg po QD *and* sulfadiazine 4-8 g po/IV QD *and* folinic acid 10 mg po QD]. *Treat for 3-6 weeks.*

Secondary prophylaxis after acute treatment of patients with AIDS

Child: [Pyrimethamine 1 mg/kg po QD *and* sulfadiazine 100 mg/kg/d (max 8 g/d) divided TID-QID *and* folinic acid 5-10 mg po QD].
Adult: [Pyrimethamine 50 mg po QD *and* sulfadiazine 2 g po QD *and* folinic acid 10 mg po QD].

Urethritis, non-gonococcal

Doxycycline 100 mg po BID or tetracycline 500 mg po QID for 7d **preferred**; *or* Erythromycin base 500 mg po QID for 7d **preferred if preg. or <9 y.o.**; *or* Erythromycin ethylsuccinate 800 mg po QID for 7d **preferred if preg. or <9 y.o.**; *Or if cannot tolerate high-dose erythromycin:* erythromycin base 250 mg po QID for 14d *or* erythromycin ethylsuccinate 400 mg po QID for 14d.

* FOR DRUG DOSING SEE TABLE BEGINNING ON PAGE 36.

Drug Therapy of Specific Disease Entities

For generic names of proprietary meds, see index

DISEASE	REGIMEN

Urinary tract infection

Cystitis

Single dose and 3d regimens only for uncomplicated UTI's in non-pregnant women. Use 7d regimens for pts with diabetes, sx >7d, recent UTI, use of diaphragm, or age >65 y.o.

Single dose
Three day

Adult: Trimethoprim/sulfa 2 DS; *or* trimeth 400 mg; *or* nitrofurantoin 200 mg.

Adult: Trimethoprim/sulfa 1 DS BID; *or* trimethoprim 100 mg BID; *or* norfloxacin 400 mg BID; *or* ciprofloxacin 250 mg BID; *or* ofloxacin 200 mg BID; *or* enoxacin 400 mg BID; *or* lomefloxacin 400 mg BID; *or* cinoxacin 500 mg po BID.

Seven day

Child: Amoxicillin*, *or* trimethoprim/sulfa*, *or* cephalexin*, *or* sulfisoxazole* .

Adult: same drugs and doses as for 3 day regimens.

Pregnant

Amoxicillin 500 mg TID; *or* cefpodoxime 100 mg BID; *or* trimethoprim/sulfa (avoid in third trimester) 2 DS BID. *Treat for 7d.*

Pyelonephritis
Outpatient

Usually women 18-40 y.o. with fever >102°F, CVA tenderness. Treat for at least 14d.

Child: Trimethoprim/sulfa*; *or* cephalexin*; *or* amoxicillin/clavulanate* .

Adult: Trimethoprim/sulfa 1 DS BID; *or* cephalexin 500 mg QID; *or* amox/clavulanate (as amox) 500 mg TID; *or* ciprofloxacin 500-750 mg BID; *or* norfloxacin 400 mg BID; *or* ofloxacin 200-400 mg BID; *or* norfloxacin 400 mg BID; *or* lomefloxacin 400 mg BID; *or* cinoxacin 500 mg BID.

Inpatient

Child/adult uncomplicated: [Gentamicin* and ampicillin*]; *or* ampicillin/sulbactam*; *or* 3rd gen ceph*; *or* trimeth/sulfa IV*; *or* piperacillin/tazobactam*; *or* carbenicillin*; *or* ticarcillin*; *or* piperacillin*; *or* mezlocillin* .

Adult complicated by obstruction, reflux, azotemia, transplant: ceftazidime*; *or* cefoperazone*; *or* [either (amikacin* *or* gentamicin* *or* tobramycin*) *and either* (carbenicillin* *or* ticarcillin* *or* piperacillin* *or* mezlocillin*)]; *or* ciprofloxacin IV; *or* ofloxacin IV.

Vaginitis

Bacterial vaginosis

Metronidazole 500 mg po BID for 7d **preferred**; *or*
Clindamycin cream 2% one full applicator intravaginally at hs for 7d **preferred if pregnant**; *or*
Metronidazole gel 0.75% one full applicator intravaginally for 5d; *or*
Clindamycin 300 mg po BID for 7d.
Do not treat sexual partners.
Diagnose if three of these found: homogeneous, white non-inflammatory discharge adherent to vaginal walls; clue cells by micro; vaginal fluid pH >4.5; fishy odor to vaginal discharge sample before or after 10% KOH.

Candida/yeast

Butoconazole 2% cream*; *or* clotrimazole 1% cream* *or* vag tabs*; *or* miconazole vag supp*; *or* terconazole 0.4%, or terconazole 6.5% ointment*; *or* tioconazole 0.4%, 0.8% cream* *or* vag supp*; *or* fluconazole 150 mg po single dose.
Mild-moderate cases: may treat with single dose; severe or complicated cases, or pregnant: 3-7d regimens.

Trichomonas

Child: Metronidazole 5 mg/kg/dose po TID for 7d.
Adult: Metronidazole 2 g po single dose or 500 mg po BID for 7d.
Treat sexual partners. If single dose therapy fails, try BID-7d regimen above.
For repeated failures: metronidazole 2 g po QD for 3-5d.

---

* *For drug dosing see table beginning on page 36.*

Drug Therapy of Specific Disease Entities

For generic names of proprietary meds, see index

DISEASE	REGIMEN

Varicella-zoster

Chicken pox

Normal host

Child 2-12 y.o.: Acyclovir 80 mg/kg/d (max 3.2 g/d) po divided QID for 5d.

Child >12 y.o.-adult: Acyclovir 800 mg po 5 times a day for 7d or 5 mg/kg IV Q8h. *Treat if: underlying skin/lung problem; on salicylates or steroids; clinically ill; >12 y.o.; pneumonia present; pregnant; or if otherwise at risk for mod-severe chicken pox.*

Immunocompromised

Child <1 y.o.: Acyclovir 30 mg/kg/d IV divided Q8h for 7-10d.

Child >1 y.o.: Acyclovir 1500 mg/m²/d IV divided Q8h for 7-10d.

Adult: Acyclovir 10-12 mg/kg IV Q8h for 7d.

Zoster

Normal host (or mild case, immunocompromised pt)

Child 12 y.o.-adult: Acyclovir 800 mg po 5 times a day for 7-10d; or famciclovir 500 mg po Q8h for 7d.

Immunocomp./severe case
(>1 dermatome, trigeminal nerve involved, disem. zoster)

Child: Acyclovir: same doses as for chicken pox immunocompromised.

Adult: Acyclovir 10-12 mg/kg IV Q8h for 7-14d. Reduce to 7.5 mg/kg/dose for older patients.

Venous thrombosis, deep

Consider thrombolytics for proximal occluding DVT.

For prophylaxis see p. 27.

Child: Heparin 50 U/kg IV, then infusion at 10-25 U/kg/h; or urokinase 4000 CTA U/kg IV over 10min, then infusion at 4000 U/kg/h for 12-24h.

Adult: Heparin 70-100 U/kg IV, then infusion at 15 U/kg/h; or urokinase 4000 CTA U/kg IV over 30min, then infusion 4000 U/kg/h for 12-24h.

Premedicate for urokinase with acetaminophen 325-650 mg po, hydrocortisone 50-100 mg IV, diphenhydramine 25-50 mg IV. After thrombolytic infusion, start heparin infusion at dose given above (omit loading dose).

Von Willebrand's disease	See p. 170.
Worms	
Hookworm (*Ancylostoma duodenale, necator americanus*)	*Child/adult:* Mebendazole 100 mg po BID for 3d; *or* pyrantel pamoate 11 mg/kg po (max 1.0 g) QD for 3d.
Pinworm (*Enterobius vermicularis*)	*Child/adult:* Pyrantel pamoate 11 mg/kg (max 1.0 g) po—repeat dose 2 weeks later; *or* mebendazole 100 mg po—repeat dose 2 weeks later.
Roundworm (*Ascaris lumbricoides*)	*Child/adult:* Mebendazole 100 mg po BID for 3d; *or* pyrantel pamoate 11 mg/kg (max 1.0 g) po single dose.
Tapeworm, beef (*Taenia saginata*)	*Child:* Praziquantel 5-10 mg/kg po single dose; *or* niclosamide 1.0 g *(11-34 kg)* or 1.5 g *(>34 kg)* po single dose. *Chew niclosamide thoroughly before swallowing.* *Adult:* Praziquantel 20 mg/kg po single dose; *or* niclosamide 2.0 g po single dose. *Chew niclosamide thoroughly before swallowing.*
Tapeworm, fish (*Diphyllobothrium lathium*)	*Child:* Praziquantel 5-10 mg/kg po single dose; *or* niclosamide 1.0 g *(11-34 kg)* or 1.5 g *(>34 kg)* po single dose. *Chew niclosamide thoroughly before swallowing.* *Adult:* Praziquantel 10 mg/kg po single dose; *or* niclosamide 2.0 g po single dose. *Chew niclosamide thoroughly before swallowing.*
Tapeworm, pork (*Taenia solium*)	*Child:* Praziquantel 5-10 mg/kg po single dose; *or* niclosamide 1.0 g *(11-34 kg)* or 1.5 g *(>34 kg)* po single dose. *Chew niclosamide thoroughly before swallowing.* *Adult:* Praziquantel 5 mg/kg po single dose; *or* niclosamide 2.0 g po single dose. *Chew niclosamide thoroughly before swallowing.*
Whipworm (*Trichuris trichiura*)	*Child/adult:* Mebendazole 100 mg po BID for 3d.

* FOR DRUG DOSING SEE TABLE BEGINNING ON PAGE 36.

Pediatric and Adult Drug Dosing

See index for generic names of proprietary meds

MEDICATION	PREPARATIONS	DOSING
Acebutolol (*Sectral*)	*Cap:* 200, 400 mg	*Adult:* **HTN:** 400-800 mg po QD or divided BID, max 1200 mg divided BID. **Ventricular arrhythmias:** start 200 mg po BID. Maintenance usually 600-1200 mg/d.
Acetaminophen (*Tylenol*)	*Drops:* 100 mg/ml *Liquid:* 120, 160, 320 mg/5 ml *Tab:* 80, 160 (*both chew*); 325, 500, 650 mg *Supp:* 120, 125, 300, 325, 650 mg	*Child:* 10-15 mg/kg/dose po Q 4-6h. *Adult:* 325-1000 mg po Q 4-6h. Max dose 4 g/d.
Acetaminophen/ codeine (*Tylenol #1, #2, #3, #4*)	*Liquid:* Acet 120 mg, codeine 12 mg/5 ml *Tab:* Acet 300 mg, codeine 7.5, 15, 30, or 60 mg	*Child:* 0.5-1.0 mg codeine/kg/dose po Q 4-6h. *Adult:* as codeine 15-60 mg po Q 4-6h.
Acetazolamide (*Diamox, Ak-Zol*)	*Tab:* 125, 250 mg *Tab (LA):* 500 mg *Inj:* 500 mg/5 ml	**Glaucoma:** *Child:* 2-7.5 mg/kg/dose po Q 6h or 5-10 mg/kg/dose IV Q 6h. *Adult:* 250-1000 mg/d po/IV divided Q 6h. **CHF:** *Child:* 5 mg/kg/dose po/IV QD. *Adult:* 250-375 mg po/IV QD.
Acetohexamide (*Dymelor*)	*Tab:* 250, 500 mg	*Adult:* 250-1500 mg po QD or divided BID.

Acetylcysteine *(Mucomyst)*	*Liquid:* 10, 20%	**Acetaminophen overdose:** *Child/adult:* 140 mg/kg po initial dose, then 70 mg/kg/dose po Q 4h for 17 doses.
Acyclovir *(Zovirax)*	*Liquid:* 200 mg/5 ml *Tab:* 800 mg *Cap:* 200 mg *Ointment:* 5% *Inj:* 500, 1000 mg/vial	**Herpes simplex:** see p. 15. **Varicella:** see p.34 .
Adenosine *(Adenocard)*	*Inj:* 6 mg/2 ml	*Child:* 0.1 mg/kg IV rapidly, repeat 0.05 mg/kg dose Q 2min IV to max 0.25 mg/kg or 12 mg total, whichever is less. *Adult:* 6 mg IV rapidly, repeat 12 mg IV Q 2min maximum twice as necessary.
Albumin	*Inj:* 5% in 50, 250, 500, 1000 ml; 25% in 20, 50, 100 ml	**Hypovolemia:** *Child:* 1 g/kg IV over 30-120min. *Adult:* 25 g IV.
Albuterol *(Proventil, Ventolin)*	*Liquid:* 2 mg/5 ml *Tab:* 2, 4 mg *Tab (SR):* 4 mg *Inhaler:* 90 µg/puff *Inhalation soltn:* 5 mg/ml; 2.5 mg/5 ml *Rotacaps:* 200 µg	**PO:** *Child <6 y.o.:* 0.1 mg/kg/dose TID, max 2 mg/dose. *Child 6-11 y.o.:* 2 mg/dose TID-QID. *Child >12 y.o.-adult:* 2-4 mg/dose TID-QID. **Inhaler:** *Child/adult:* 1-2 puffs Q 4-6h prn. **Nebulized:** *Child:* 0.10-0.15 mg/kg/dose (max 5 mg) in 2 ml NS Q 4h. *Adult:* 2.5-5.0 mg in 2 ml NS Q 4h. **Rotacaps:** *Child >4 y.o.-adult:* 200 µg Q 4-6h via Rotahaler.
Allopurinol *(Zyloprim)*	*Tab:* 100, 300 mg	*Child:* 10 mg/kg/d po divided TID-QID, max 600 mg/d. *Adult:* 100-800 mg/d QD or in divided doses.

Pediatric and Adult Drug Dosing

See index for generic names of proprietary meds

MEDICATION	PREPARATIONS	DOSING
Alprazolam (*Xanax*)	*Tab:* 0.25, 0.5, 1, 2 mg	*Adult:* 0.25-1 mg po TID.
Alteplase (*Activase*)	*Inj:* 1 mg/ml in 20, 50, 100 ml vials	**Acute MI/pulmonary embolism:** *Adult <65 kg:* 0.125 mg/kg IV over 1-2min, then 0.625 mg/kg over 1h, then 0.25 mg/kg/h IV for 2h, total dose 1.25 mg/kg. *Adult >65 kg:* 10 mg over 1-2min, then 50 mg IV over 1h, then 20 mg/h for 2h.
Aluminum hydroxide (*Alternajel, Alu-Cap, Alu-Tab, Amphojel*)	*Liquid:* 600 mg (Alternajel); 320 mg/5 ml (Amphojel) *Cap:* 475 mg (Alu-Cap); 500 mg (Dialume) *Tab:* 600 mg (Alu-Tab); 300, 600 mg (Amphojel)	**Antacid:** *Child/adult: Liquid:* 500-1800 mg (5-15 ml) po after meals and at hs. *Tab:* 300-600 mg chew before swallowing with milk or water after meals and at hs. *Cap:* 1-3 po after meals and at hs. **Hyperphosphatemia in chronic renal failure:** *Child/adult:* 2.0 g/dose po BID-QID.
Amantidine (*Symmetrel*)	*Cap:* 100 mg *Liquid:* 50 mg/5 ml	**Influenza A:** *Child 1-9 y.o.:* 1.1-2.2 mg/kg/dose po BID. *Child >9 y.o.-adult:* 200 mg/d po QD or divided BID. **Parkinson's:** *Adult:* 100 mg po BID; if seriously ill or receiving other anti-Parkinsonian drugs, 100 mg po QD for at least 1wk, then 100 mg po BID as needed.
Amikacin (*Amikin*)	*Inj:* 50, 250 mg/ml	**IM/IV:** *Child <7 days:* initial dose 10 mg/kg, then 7.5 mg/kg/dose Q12h. *Child >7 days:* 15 mg/kg/d divided Q8-12h. *Adult:* 10 mg/kg load, then 7.5 mg Q12h. *Alternate QD dosing (adult only):* 15 mg/kg IV only.

Drug	Forms	Dosing
Amiloride (*Midamor*)	*Tab:* 5 mg	*Child:* 0.625 mg/kg/dose po QD. *Adult:* 5-20 mg po QD.
Aminophylline	*Liquid:* 105 mg/5 ml *Tab:* 100, 200 mg *Tab (LA):* 225 mg *Rect supp:* 250, 500 mg *Inj:* 25 mg/ml	**PO:** *Child 1-9 y.o.:* 20 mg/kg/d divided Q 4-6h. *Child 9-16 y.o.:* 4 mg/kg/dose Q 6h. *Child >16 y.o.-adult:* 3 mg/kg/dose Q 6h. **IV load:** *Child/adult:* 6 mg/kg lean body weight over 20min. **IV maintenance:** *Neonates:* 0.2 mg/kg/h. *6 wk-6 mo.:* 0.5 mg/kg/h. *6 mo.-1 y.o.:* 0.6-0.7 mg/kg/h. *1-9 y.o.:* 1.0-1.2 mg/kg/h. *9-12 y.o, and young adult smokers:* 0.9 mg/kg/h. Adult non-smokers: 0.7 mg/kg/h. Adult smokers: 1 mg/kg/h. Adult, older, or with cor pulmonale: 0.6 mg/kg/h for 12h, then 0.3 mg/kg/h. Adult w CHF/liver disease: 0.5 mg/kg/h for 12h, then 0.1-0.2 mg/h.
Amiodarone (*Cordarone*)	*Tab:* 200 mg	**PO:** *Adult:* 800-1600 mg QD for 1-3wk, then 600-800 mg QD for 4wk, then 200-400 mg QD. Divide doses for side effects.
Amitriptyline (*Elavil, Endep*)	*Tab:* 10, 25, 50, 75, 100, 150 mg	*Maintenance: Adolescents:* 100-300 mg/d divided BID-TID. *Adult:* 50-100 mg QD.
Amlodipine (*Norvasc*)	*Tab:* 2.5, 5, 10 mg	*Adult: HTN:* 2.5-10 mg po QD. *Angina:* 5-10 mg QD.
Amoxapine (*Asendin*)	*Tab:* 25, 50, 100, 150 mg	*Maintenance: Adult:* 100-300 mg/d po divided BID-TID.
Amoxicillin (*Amox, Polymox, Trimox, Ultimox, Wymox*)	*Liquid:* 50, 125, 250 mg/5 ml *Tab (chew):* 125, 250 mg *Cap:* 250, 500 mg	*Child:* 7-13 mg/kg/dose po Q 8h. *Adult:* 250-500 mg po Q 8h.

Pediatric and Adult Drug Dosing

See index for generic names of proprietary meds

MEDICATION	PREPARATIONS	DOSING
Amoxicillin/ clavulanate *(Augmentin)*	*Liquid:* A 125 mg, C 31.25 mg/5 ml; A 250 mg, C 62.5 mg/5 ml *Tab (chew):* A 125 mg, C 31.25 mg; A 250 mg, C 62.5 mg *Tab:* A 250 mg, C 125 mg; A 500 mg, C 125 mg	*Child:* as amoxicillin 7-13 mg/kg/dose po Q 8h. *Adult:* as amoxicillin 250-500 mg po Q 8h.
Ampicillin *(Amcil, Omnipen, Polycillin, Principen, Roampicillin, Totacillin)*	*Liquid:* 100, 125, 250, 500 mg/5 ml *Cap:* 250, 500 mg *Inj:* 125, 250, 500, 1000, 2000 mg/dose	**PO:** *Child:* 12-25 mg/kg/dose Q 6h. *Adult:* 250-500 mg Q 6h. **IM/IV:** *Child <7 days:* **Meningitis:** 50 mg/kg/dose IV Q 12h. *Child <7 days:* **Other:** 25 mg/kg/dose IM/IV Q 12h. *Child >7 d:* **Meningitis:** 38-50 mg/kg/dose IV Q 6h. *Child >7 days:* **Other:** 25 mg/kg/dose IM/IV Q 8h. *Adult:* **Meningitis:** 2 g IV Q 4h. *Adult:* **Other:** 1-2 g IV Q 4-6h.
Ampicillin/ sulbactam *(Unasyn)*	*Inj:* Amp 1.5 g, Sul 0.5 g; Amp 3.0 g, Sul 1 g	*Child >12 y.o.-adult:* As ampicillin: 1.5-3.0 g IM/IV Q 6h.
Anistreplase *(Eminase)*	*Inj:* 30 units/vial	**Acute MI:** *Adult:* 30 U IV over 2-5min.
Antipyrine/benzocaine *(Auralgan)*	*Otic sltn:* Antipyrine 5.4%, Benzo 1.4%	**Acute OM:** *Child/adult:* fill external ear canal Q 1-2h prn. **Cerumen impaction:** fill canal TID for 2-3d prior to cerumen removal.

Aspirin	*Tab:* 81 mg *(chew),* 165, 325, 500, 650, 975 mg *Supp:* 65, 120, 130, 195, 200, 300, 325, 600, 650 mg	*Child:* 10-15 mg/kg/dose po Q 4h. *Adult:* varies with disease.
Astemizole *(Hismanal)*	*Tab:* 10 mg	*Child 6-12 y.o:* 5 mg po QD. *Child 12 y.o.-adult:* 10 mg po QD.
Atenolol *(Tenormin)*	*Tab:* 50, 100 mg	*Adult:* 50-100 mg po QD.
Atovaquone *(Mepron)*	*Tab:* 250 mg	*Pneumocystis pneumonia:* see p. 24.
Atracurium *(Tracrium)*	*Inj:* 10 mg/ml	*Initial: Child 1 mo.-2 y.o.:* 0.3-0.4 mg/kg/dose IV push. *Child >2 y.o.-adult:* 0.4-0.5 mg/kg/dose IV push. *Maintenance of paralysis: Child/adult:* only after evidence of recovery from initial dose give 9-10 μg/kg/min until spontaneous recovery halted, then 5-9 μg/kg/min. Dose range is 2-15 μg/kg/min to maintain paralysis.
Atropine	*Inj:* 0.05, 0.1, 0.3, 0.4, 0.5, 0.8, 1.0 mg/ml	*Heart block: Child:* 0.01-0.03 mg/kg/dose IV/ET. *Minimum dose 0.1 mg, max 1.0 mg.* *Adult:* 0.5-1.0 mg IV/ET Q 5min. Max total dose 3 mg. *Asystole: Adult:* 1.0 mg initially, repeat Q 5min prn. *Bronchospasm: Child:* 0.05 mg/kg/dose (0.25-1.0 mg) with 2 ml NS nebulized. *Adult:* 2-3 mg in 2 ml nebulized Q 6h. *Reversal of non-depolarizing paralyzing agents:* *Child:* 0.01 mg/kg/dose, give with neostigmine. Min dose 0.1 mg. *Adult:* 0.5 mg/dose, give with neostigmine.

Pediatric and Adult Drug Dosing

See index for generic names of proprietary meds

MEDICATION	PREPARATIONS	DOSING
Azithromycin (*Zithromax*)	*Cap:* 250 mg	***COPD, pneumonia, cellulitis:*** *Child >16 y.o.-adult:* 500 mg po once on day 1, then 250 mg QD days 2 to 5. ***Chancroid:*** see p. 8. ***Chlamydia:*** see p. 8.
Aztreonam (*Azactam*)	*Inj:* 0.5, 1, 2 g	IV: *Child >1 mo.:* 30 mg/kg/dose Q6h. *Adult:* 1-2 g Q6-8h.
Baclofen (*Lioresal*)	*Tab:* 10, 20 mg	PO: *Child >2 y.o.:* 3.3-5 mg/kg/dose TID, max 2-7 y.o., 40 mg/d; max >7 y.o., 60 mg/d. *Adult:* start 5 mg po TID, increase by 5 mg po TID Q 3d until desired effect attained. Max dose 20 mg TID-QID.
Beclomethasone (*Vanceril, Beclovent, Beconase*)	*Inhaler:* 42 µg/puff *Nasal spray:* 42 µg/spray	**Inhaler:** *Child 6-12 y.o.:* 1-2 puffs Q6-8h, max 10 puffs/d. *Child >12 y.o.-adult:* 2-4 puffs Q6-8h, max 20 puffs/d. **Nasal spray:** *Child 6-12 y.o.:* 1 spray each nostril TID. *Child 12 y.o.-adult:* 2 sprays each nostril BID.
Benazepril (*Lotensin*)	*Tab:* 5, 10, 20, 40 mg	PO: *Adult:* 10-40 mg/d QD or divided BID.
Benztropine mesylate (*Cogentin*)	*Tab:* 0.5, 1, 2 mg *Inj:* 1 mg/ml	***Dystonic reaction:*** *Adult:* 1 mg IV/IM, then 1-2 mg po BID for 3d.
Bepridil (*Vascor*)	*Tab:* 200, 300, 400 mg	PO: *Adult:* 200-400 mg QD.

Betaxolol *(Kerlone)*	*Tab:* 10, 20 mg	**PO:** *Adult:* 10-20 mg QD.
Bethanecol *(Urecholine, Duvoid)*	*Tab:* 5, 10, 25, 50 mg *Inj:* 5 mg/ml	**PO:** *Adult:* 10-50 mg TID-QID. **SQ:** *Adult:* 2.5 mg Q 15min prn up to 4 doses, then give sum of initial doses Q 6h. *Never give IV or IM.*
Bicarbonate, sodium	*Inj:* 44, 50 mEq/50 ml; 5, 10 mEq/10 ml; 2.5 mEq/5 ml	**CPR:** *Child/adult:* 1 mEq/kg IV Q 10min. Use solution of 0.5 mEq/ml for neonates, 1 mEq/ml for others.
Bisacodyl *(Dulcolax)*	*Tab:* 5 mg *Supp:* 10 mg	*Child:* 1-2 tabs po QD; or ½ supp PR QD if age <2 y.o., 1 supp PR QD if >2 y.o. *Adult:* 10-15 mg po or PR QD.
Bisoprolol fumarate *(Zebeta)*	*Tab:* 5, 10 mg	*Adult:* 5-20 mg po QD.
Bitolterol *(Tornalate)*	*Inhaler:* 370 μg/puff	*Child >12 y.o.-adult:* 2-3 puffs Q 6-8h.
Bretylium *(Bretylol)*	*Inj:* 50 mg/ml	*Child >12 y.o.-adult:* initial dose 5 mg/kg/dose IV, then 5-10 mg/kg/dose IV Q 15-30min, max total 30 mg/kg. Infusion 1-2 mg/min.
Bumetanide *(Bumex)*	*Tab:* 0.5, 1, 2 mg *Inj:* 0.25 mg/ml	**PO:** *Child >6 mo.:* 0.02-0.1 mg/kg/dose QD or QOD. *Adult:* 0.5-2 mg/d QD. **IM/IV:** *Child >6 mo.:* 0.02-0.1 mg/kg/dose. *Adult:* 0.5-1.0 mg over 1-2min; may repeat Q 2h, max 10 mg/d.

Pediatric and Adult Drug Dosing

See index for generic names of proprietary meds

MEDICATION	PREPARATIONS	DOSING
Buspirone (*BuSpar*)	*Tab:* 5, 10 mg	*Adult:* start 5 mg po TID. Dose may be increased by 5 mg/d every 2-3d. Max 60 mg/d.
Butoconazole (*Femstat*)	*Cream:* 2%	*Vaginal candidiasis:* one applicator full Q hs for 3-6d.
Butorphanol (*Stadol*)	*Inj:* 1, 2 mg/ml *Nasal:* 10 mg/ml	**IM:** *Adult:* 1-4 mg Q 3-4h prn. **IV:** *Adult:* 0.5-2.0 mg Q 3-4h prn. **Nasal:** *Adult:* 1-2 mg (1-2 sprays) Q 3-4h prn.
Calcium chloride	*Inj:* 100 mg (1.36 mEq)/ml in 10 ml	*Child:* 20 mg (0.2 ml)/kg/dose IV Q 10min prn. *Adult:* 250-500 mg (2.5-5.0 ml)/dose IV Q 10min prn.
Calcium gluconate	*Inj:* 100 mg (0.45mEq)/ml in 10 ml	*Child:* 50-100 mg (1.0 ml)/kg/dose IV Q 10min prn. *Adult:* 0.5-1.0 g (5-10 ml)/dose IV Q 10min prn. *Calcium chloride generally preferred.*
Calcitriol (*Rocalcitrol*)	*Cap:* 0.25, 0.5 μg	*Adult:* 0.25 μg po QOD up to 1.25 μg po QD.
Capsaicin (*Zostrix*)	*Cream:* 0.025%, 0.075%	*Child >2 y.o.:* apply to affected area of skin TID-QID.
Captopril (*Capoten*)	*Tab:* 12.5, 25, 50, 100 mg	**HTN:** *Child <1 mo.:* 0.01 mg/kg/dose po Q 6-12h. *Child >1 mo.-12 y.o.:* start 0.3 mg/kg/dose po TID. May increase every 8-24h by 0.3 mg/kg/dose. If on diuretics, has renal impairment, or is volume depleted, start at 0.15 mg/kg/dose. *Child >12 y.o.-adult:* start 25 mg/dose po BID-TID. Increase Q 2wk as needed to max 450 mg/d divided BID-TID.

Drug	Forms	Dosing
Carbamazepine (Tegretol)	Liquid: 100 mg/5 ml Tab: 100 (chew), 200 mg	**CHF:** *Child <1 mo.:* 0.1-0.4 mg/kg/d po divided Q 6-8h. *Child >1 mo.-1 y.o.:* 0.5-0.6 mg/kg/d po divided Q 6-12h. *Child >1 y.o.-12 y.o.:* 12.5 mg/dose po Q 12h. *Adult:* start 25 mg po TID, may increase to max 150 mg po Q 8h. If on diuretic start at 6.25-12.5 mg po TID. **Seizure loading dose:** *Child <12 y.o.:* liquid 10 mg/kg po. *Child >12 y.o.-adult:* liquid 8 mg/kg po. **Seizure maintenance:** *Child <6 y.o.:* 5-20 mg/kg/d po divided Q 6-8h. *Child 6-12 y.o.:* 20-30 mg/kg/d po divided Q 6-8h. *Child 12-15 y.o.:* 400-1000 mg/d po divided Q 6-8h. *Child 15 y.o.-adult:* 400-1200 mg/d po divided Q 6-8h.
Carbenicillin (Geocillin)	Tab: 382 mg	*Adult:* 1-2 tabs po Q 6h.
Carisoprodol (Soma)	Tab: 350 mg	*Adult:* 350 mg po Q 6h.
Carteolol (Cartrol)	Tab: 2.5, 5 mg	*Adult:* 2.5-10 mg po QD.
Cefaclor (2nd gen) (Ceclor)	Liquid: 125, 187, 250, 375 mg/5 ml Cap: 250, 500 mg	*Child:* **Acute otitis media:** 13.3 mg/kg/dose po TID. **Other:** 7.3 mg/kg/dose TID. Max 1 g/d. *Adult:* 250-500 mg/dose po Q 8h.
Cefadroxil (1st gen) (Duricef, Ultracef)	Liquid: 125, 250, 500 mg/5 ml Cap: 500 mg Tab: 1 g	*Child:* 15 mg/kg/dose po Q 12h. *Adult:* 0.5-1.0 g/dose po Q 12h.

Pediatric and Adult Drug Dosing

See index for generic names of proprietary meds

MEDICATION	PREPARATIONS	DOSING
Cefamandole (*2nd gen*) (*Mandol*)	*Inj*: 0.5, 1, 2, 10 g	*Child >1 mo.*: 50-150 mg/kg/d IM/IV divided Q4-6h. *Adult*: 0.5-2.0 g IM/IV 4-6h.
Cefazolin (*1st gen*) (*Ancef, Kefzol*)	*Inj*: 0.25, 0.5, 0.5, 1, 5, 10 g	*Child <7 days*: 20 mg/kg/dose IM/IV Q 12h. *Child >7 days*: 13.3 mg/kg/dose IM/IV Q 8h. *Adult*: 0.25-1.5 g IM/IV Q 6-8h.
Cefixime (*3rd gen*) (*Suprax*)	*Liquid*: 100 mg/5 ml *Tab*: 200, 400 mg	*Child*: 8 mg/kg/dose po QD. *Adult*: 400 mg po QD.
Cefmetazole (*2nd gen*) (*Zefazone*)	*Inj*: 1, 2 g	*Adult*: 2 g IV Q 6-12h.
Cefonicid (*2nd gen*) (*Monocid*)	*Inj*: 0.5, 1.0 g	*Adult*: 1-2 g IM/IV QD.
Cefoperazone (*3rd gen*) (*Cefobid*)	*Inj*: 1, 2 g	*Child <1 mo.*: 50 mg/kg/dose IV Q 12h. *Child >1 mo.*: 37.5 mg/kg/dose IV Q 6h. *Adult*: **Pyelonephritis** 1 g IV Q 12h. **Other**: 2-4 g IV Q 6-12h.
Cefotaxime (*3rd gen*) (*Claforan*)	*Inj*: 0.5, 1.0, 2.0 g	*Child all ages*: **Meningitis**: 50 mg/kg/dose IV Q 6h, max 12 g/d. *Child <7 days*: **Other**: 50 mg/kg/dose IV Q 12h. *Child >7 days*: **Other**: 50 mg/kg/dose IV Q 8h. *Adult*: **Meningitis**: 2 g IV Q 4h. *Adult*: **Other**: 1-2 g IM/IV Q 4-12h.

Cefotetan (*2nd gen*) (*Cefotan*)	*Inj:* 1, 2 g	*Adult:* 1-3 g IM/IV Q12h, max 6 g/d.
Cefoxitin (*2nd gen*) (*Mefoxin*)	*Inj:* 1, 2 g	*Child < 7 days:* 20 mg/kg/dose IM/IV Q12h. *Child > 7 days:* 20-40 mg/kg/dose IM/IV Q 6h, max 12g/d. *Adult:* 1-2 g/dose IM/IV Q4-8h.
Cefpodoxime (*3rd gen*) (*Vantin*)	*Liquid:* 50, 100 mg/5 ml *Tab:* 100, 200 mg	*Child >6 mo.: **Otitis media:*** 5 mg/kg/dose Q12h. *Adult: **UTI:*** 100 mg Q12h for 7d. ***Other:*** 200-400 mg Q12h for 7-14d.
Cefprozil (*2nd gen*) (*Cefzil*)	*Liquid:* 125, 250 mg/ml *Tab:* 250, 500 mg	*Child >6 mo.:* 15 mg/kg/dose po BID. *Adult:* 500 mg po BID.
Ceftazidime (*3rd gen*) (*Fortaz, Tazicef, Tazidime*)	*Inj:* 1, 2 g	*Child <1 mo.:* 30 mg/kg/dose IV Q 12h. *Child >1 mo.:* 50 mg/kg/dose IV Q 8h, max 6 g/d. *Adult: **Meningitis:*** 2-3 g IV Q8h. *Adult: **Other:*** 1-2 g IM/IV Q8-12h.
Ceftizoxime (*3rd gen*) (*Cefizox*)	*Inj:* 1, 2 g	*Child:* 50-67 mg/kg/dose IV Q8h. *Adult: **Meningitis:*** 2-3 g IV Q8h. *Adult: **Other:*** 1-4 g IM/IV Q8-12h.
Ceftriaxone (*3rd gen*) (*Rocephin*)	*Inj:* 0.25, 0.5, 1.0, 2.0 g	*Child: **Meningitis:*** initial dose 75 mg/kg IV, then 50 mg/kg/dose IV Q12h. *Child: **Other:*** 50 mg/kg/dose IM/IV Q 24h. *Adult: **Meningitis:*** 2-3 g IV Q12h. *Adult: **Other:*** 1-2 g IM/IV Q24h.

Pediatric and Adult Drug Dosing

See index for generic names of proprietary meds

MEDICATION	PREPARATIONS	DOSING
Cefuroxime (*2nd gen*) (*Ceftin, Kefurox, Zinacef*)	*Tab*: 125, 250, 500 mg *Inj*: 0.75, 1.5 g	**PO**: *Child*: *Otitis media*: 20 mg/kg/dose po BID. *Other*: 15 mg/kg/dose po BID. *Adult*: 250-500 mg BID. **IM/IV**: *Child >3 mo.*: **Meningitis**: 50-60 mg/kg/dose IV Q 6h. *Child >3 mo.*: *Other*: 25 mg/kg/dose IV Q 8h. *Adult*: 0.75-1.5 g IM/IV Q 8h.
Cephalexin (*1st gen*) (*Keflex, Keftab, Keflet*)	*Liquid*: 125, 250 mg/5 ml *Cap*: 250, 500 mg *Tab*: 250, 500 mg	*Child*: 6-12 mg/kg/dose po Q 6h. *Adult*: 250-1000 mg po Q 6h.
Cephalothin (*1st gen*) (*Keflin, Seffin*)	*Inj*: 1, 2 g	*Child*: 13-26 mg/kg/dose IV Q 4h. *Adult*: 0.5-2.0 g IV Q 4-6h.
Cephapirin (*1st gen*) (*Cefadyl*)	*Inj*: 0.5, 1.0, 2.0 g	*Child >3 mo*: 10-20 mg/kg/dose IV Q 6h. *Adult*: 0.5-2.0 g IV Q 4-6h.
Cephradine (*1st gen*) (*Velosef, Anspor*)	*Liquid*: 125, 250 mg/5 ml *Cap*: 250, 500 mg *Inj*: 0.25, 0.5, 1.0, 2.0, 4.0 g	**PO**: *Child*: 25-50 mg/kg/d divided Q 6-12h, max 4 g/d. *Adult*: 250-1000 mg Q 6h. **IM/IV**: *Child >1 y.o.*: 50-100 mg/kg/d divided Q 6-12h. *Adult*: 0.5-2.0 g Q 4-6h.
Chloral hydrate	*Liquid*: 250, 500 mg/5 ml *Cap*: 250, 500 mg *Supp*: 324, 500, 648 mg	**PO/PR**: *Hypnotic dose*: *Child*: 50-75 mg/kg/dose (max 1 g/dose or 2 g/d). *Adult*: 500-1000 mg/dose (max 1 g/dose or max 2 g/d).

Chloramphenicol (*Chloromycetin*)	*Inj:* 1, 10 g	**IV:** *Child <7 days:* 25 mg/kg/dose QD. *Child 7 days-1 y.o.:* 25 mg/kg/dose Q 12h. *Child >1 y.o.:* **Meningitis:** 25 mg/kg/dose Q 6h. *Child >1 y.o.:* **Other:** 12.5-19 mg/kg/dose Q 6h. *Adult:* **Meningitis:** 1.0-1.5 g Q 6h. *Adult:* **Other:** 12.5 mg/kg/dose Q 6h.
Chlordiazepoxide (*Librium*)	*Cap:* 5, 10, 25 mg *Inj:* 100 mg/vial	**PO:** *Child > 6 y.o.:* 5-10 mg/dose BID-TID. *Adult:* 5-25 mg/dose BID-QID. **IM/IV:** *Adult:* 50-100 mg/dose.
Chlordiazepoxide/ clidinium (*Librax*)	*Tab:* Chlor 5 mg, Clid 2.5 mg	*Adult:* 1-2 tabs po before meals and at hs.
Chlorothiazide (*Diuril*)	*Liquid:* 250 mg/ml *Tab:* 250, 500 mg *Inj:* 40 mg/ml	*Child < 6 mo:* 10-20 mg/kg/dose po/IV Q 12h. *Child >6 mo:* 10 mg/kg/dose po/IV Q 12h. *Adult:* 0.5-2 g/d po/IV divided Q 12-24h.
Chlorpheniramine (*Chlor-Trimeton*)	*Liquid:* 2 mg/5 ml *Tab:* 2 mg (chew), 4 mg *SR cap or tab:* 6, 8, 12 mg	*Child 2-6 y.o.:* 1 mg po Q 4-6h. *Child 6-12 y.o.:* 2 mg po Q 4-6h. *Child >12 y.o.-adult:* 4 mg po Q 4-6h or SR: 8-12 mg po Q 12h.

Pediatric and Adult Drug Dosing

See index for generic names of proprietary meds

MEDICATION	PREPARATIONS	DOSING
Chlorpromazine (*Thorazine*)	*Liquid:* 30, 100 mg/ml; 10 mg/5 ml *Tab:* 10, 25, 50, 100, 200 mg *Cap:* 30, 75, 150 mg *Supp:* 25, 100 mg *Inj:* 25 mg/ml	***Nausea/vomiting: PO:*** *Child >6 mo.:* 0.55 mg/kg/dose Q 4-6h. *Adult:* 10-25 mg Q 4-6h. **PR:** *Child >6 mo.:* 1.1 mg/kg/dose Q 6-8h. *Adult:* 50-100 mg Q 6-8h. **IM:** *Child >6 mo.:* 0.55 mg/kg/dose Q 6-8h. *Adult:* 10-25 mg Q 4-6h. ***Agitation in psychotic patients:*** **IM:** *Child >6 mo.:* 0.25 mg/kg/dose Q 6-8h. *Adult:* initial dose 25 mg, may repeat 25-50 mg in 1h prn. ***Psychosis: PO:*** *Child >6 mo.:* 0.55 mg/kg/dose Q 4-6h, max 40 mg/d if <5 y.o., max 75 mg/d if 5-12 y.o. *Adult:* 30-200 mg/d divided BID-QID.
Chlorpropamide (*Diabinese*)	*Tab:* 100, 250 mg	*Adult:* 100-750 mg/d po QD.
Chlorthalidone (*Hygroton*)	*Tab:* 25, 50, 100 mg	*Child:* 2 mg/kg/dose po three times a week. *Adult:* 25-200 mg po QD.
Chlorzoxazone (*Parafon Forte*)	*Tab:* 250, 500 mg	*Child:* 5 mg/kg/dose po Q 6-8h. *Adult:* 250-750 mg po Q 6-8h.
Cholestyramine (*Questran*)	*Powder:* 5 g and 9 g packs, each contains 4 g of drug	*Child:* 240 mg/kg/d po divided TID. *Dose in g of drug.* *Adult:* 4 g (1 pack) 1-6 times/d. *Dose in g of drug.*

Cimetidine *(Tagamet)*	*Liquid:* 300 mg/5 ml *Tab:* 200, 300, 400, 800 mg *Inj:* 150 mg/ml	*Child <1 y.o.:* **PO/IM/IV:** 2.5-5.0 mg/kg/dose Q 6h. *Child >1 y.o.:* **PO/IM/IV:** 5-10 mg/kg/dose Q 6h. *Adult:* **PO:** 800 mg Q hs, or 400 mg BID, or 300 mg Q 6h. **IM/IV:** 300 mg Q 6h.
Cinoxacin *(Cinobac)*	*Cap:* 250, 500 mg	**UTI:** *Adult >18 y.o.:* 1 g/d po divided BID or QID.
Ciprofloxacin *(Cipro)*	*Tab:* 250, 500, 750 mg *Inj:* 200, 400 mg	**PO:** *Adult >18 y.o.:* 250-750 mg po BID. **GC:** see p. 13. **UTI:** see p. 32. **IV:** *Adult >18 y.o.:* 200-400 mg Q12h. *400 mg IV = 750 mg po*
Cisapride *(Propulsid)*	*Tab:* 10, 20 mg	*Adult:* 10-20 mg po QID 15min before meals and at hs.
Clarithromycin *(Biaxin)*	*Tab:* 250, 500 mg	*Child:* 7.5 mg/kg/dose (max 500 mg) po BID. *Adult:* 250-500 mg po BID.
Clindamycin *(Cleocin)*	*Liquid:* 75 mg/5 ml *Cap:* 75, 150 mg *Inj:* 150, 300, 600 mg	**PO:** *Child:* 2.0-6.3 mg/kg/dose Q 6h. *Adult:* 150-450 mg Q 6h. **IM/IV:** *Child <1 mo.:* 15-20 mg/kg/d divided Q 6-8h. *Child >1 mo.:* 20-40 mg/kg/d divided Q 6-8h. *Adult:* 150-900 mg Q 6h.
Clonazepam *(Klonopin)*	*Tab:* 0.5, 1, 2 mg	***Seizure maintenance:*** *Child:* 0.003-0.015 mg/kg/dose Q 8h. *Adult:* 0.5-6.5 mg po Q 6h.
Clonidine *(Catapres)*	*Tab:* 0.1, 0.2, 0.3 mg *Patch:* TTS-1, TTS-2, TTS-3	*Adult:* 0.1-1.2 mg BID. Patches Q wk. Patches deliver, respectively, 0.1, 0.2, 0.3 mg/d.

Pediatric and Adult Drug Dosing

See index for generic names of proprietary meds

MEDICATION	PREPARATIONS	DOSING
Clorazepate (*Tranxene*)	*Tab*: 11.25, 22.5 mg *Tab/cap*: 3.75, 7.5, 15 mg *Tab (SR)*: 11.25, 22.5 mg	***Seizure maintenance:*** *Child 9-12 y.o.*: 3.75-30 mg po BID. *Child >12 y.o.-adult*: 3.75-30 mg/dose po TID. ***Anxiety:*** *Adult*: 15-60 mg/d po divided BID-TID or (SR) 11.25-22.5 mg po QD.
Clotrimazole (*Lotrimin, Mycelex*)	*Tab (vag)*: 100, 500 mg *Oral troche*: 10 mg *Lotion, cream, sltn*: 1%	***Vaginal candidiasis:*** in vagina Q hs for 1d (500 mg), 3d (two 100 mg tabs), or 7d (100 mg). ***Thrush/candida esophagitis:*** *Child >3 y.o.-adult*: 1 troche dissolved slowly in mouth 5 times a day for 14d. ***Tinea corporis, cruris, pedis and cutaneous candidiasis:*** apply cream BID for 2-3 wks.
Cloxacillin (*Cloxapen, Tegopen*)	*Liquid*: 125 mg/ml *Cap*: 250, 500 mg	*Child*: 12-25 mg/kg/dose po Q 6h. *Adult*: 250-500 mg po Q6h.
Codeine	*Liquid*: 15 mg/5 ml *Tab*: 15, 30, 60 mg	*Child*: 0.5-1.0 mg/kg/dose po Q 4-6h. *Adult*: 15-60 mg po Q 4-6h.
Colchicine	*Tab*: 0.5, 0.6 mg *Inj*: 1 mg/2 ml	***Gout maintenance:*** *Adult*: 0.5-0.6 mg po QD. ***Acute gout attack:*** see p. 14.
Colestipol (*Colestid*)	*Packet*: Granules 5 g *Bottle*: Granules 500 g	*Child*: 500 mg/kg/d po divided BID-QID. *Adult*: 15-30 g/d po divided BID-QID.
Cromolyn sodium (*Intal, Nasalcrom*)	*Inhaler*: 800 µg/puff *Inhalation sltn*: 20 mg/2 ml	***Asthma prevention:*** *Children >5 y.o.-adult*: 2 sprays from inhaler as needed up to QID.

	Nasal sltn: 5.2 mg per metered spray	***Allergic rhinitis:*** *Children >5 y.o.-adult:* 1 spray in each nostril 3-6 times/d.
Crotamiton *(Eurax)*	*Cream, lotion:* 10%	***Scabies:*** see p. 28.
Cyclobenzaprine *(Flexeril)*	*Tab:* 10 mg	*Adult:* 20-60 mg/d po divided Q 8-12h.
Cyproheptadine *(Periactin)*	*Liquid:* 2 mg/5 ml *Tab:* 4 mg	*Child 2-6 y.o.:* 1.3-4.0 mg/dose po TID. *Child 7-14 y.o.:* 2.7-5.3 mg/dose po TID. *Child >15 y.o.-adult:* 4.0-10.7 mg/dose po TID.
Dapsone	*Tab:* 25, 100 mg	***Pneumocystis prophylaxis:*** see p. 25.
Deferoxamine *(Desferol, Mesylate)*	*Inj:* 500 mg	***Iron OD:*** *Child/adult:* 15 mg/kg/h infusion, max 6 g/24h. See p. 130.
Dexamethasone *(Decadron)*	*Elixir:* 0.5 mg/5 ml *Oral sltn:* 0.1, 1.0 mg/ml *Tab:* 0.25, 0.5, 0.75, 1.0 1.5, 2, 4, 6 mg *Inj:* 4, 8, 10, 16, 20, 24 mg/ml	*Dosage dependent on disease process undergoing treatment.*
Dextrose	*Inj:* 0.5 g/ml (D50)	*Child:* 1 ml/kg/dose IV of D50 diluted 1:1 w sterile H2O. *Adult:* 1 amp IV (= 50 ml volume = 25 g dextrose).
Diazepam *(Valium)*	*Liquid:* 1, 5 mg/ml *Tab:* 2, 5, 10 mg *Tab (SR):* 15 mg *Inj:* 5 mg/ml	**PO:** *Child >1 mo.:* 0.03-0.2 mg/kg/dose Q 6h. *Adult:* 2-10 mg Q 6-12h (SR: 15-30 mg QD). **IV:** *Child >1 mo.:* 0.25 mg/kg/dose Q 15min prn. *Adult:* 5-10 mg Q 10min prn.

Pediatric and Adult Drug Dosing

See index for generic names of proprietary meds

MEDICATION	PREPARATIONS	DOSING
Dichlorphenamide (*Daranide*)	*Tab:* 50 mg	Adult: ***Loading dose:*** 100-200 mg po, then 100 mg Q 12h to desired response. ***Maintenance:*** 25-50 mg po QD-TID.
Diclofenac (*Voltaren*)	*Tab:* 25, 50, 75 mg	Adult: 100-200 mg/d po divided Q 8-12h.
Dicloxacillin (*Dynapen*)	*Liquid:* 62.5 mg/5 ml *Cap:* 125, 250, 500 mg	Child: 12.5-50 mg/kg/d po divided Q 4-6h. Adult: 250-500 mg/dose po Q 6h.
Dicyclomine (*Bentyl*)	*Liquid:* 10 mg/5 ml *Cap:* 10, 20 mg *Tab:* 20 mg *Inj:* 10 mg/ml	Adult: **PO:** 20-40 mg Q 6h. **IM:** 20 mg Q 6h.
Didanosine (*Videx*) † *Chew tabs thoroughly or dissolve in 1 oz. water. Dissolve powder in at least 1 oz. water.* * *See p. 165 for body surface area determination.*	*Liquid:* 10 mg/ml *Tab†:* 25, 50, 100, 150 mg *Single dose packets†:* 100, 167, 250, 375 mg	*Tabs (doses in plain type) are equal to 0.8 mg of powder or liquid (doses in bold type) in mg.* Child: (by body surface area in m²*) <0.4: 25 (**30**) mg; 0.5-0.7: 50 (**60**) mg; 0.8-1.0: 75 (**95**) mg; 1.1-1.4: 100 (**125**) mg. *Take these doses BID.* Adult: 35-49 kg: 125 (**167**) mg; 50-74 kg: 200 (**250**) mg; >75 kg: 300 (**375**) mg. *Take these doses BID.*
Diflunisal (*Dolobid*)	*Tab:* 250, 500 mg	Adult: 250-500 mg po BID. Adult >70 y.o.: start with ½ usual dose.

Digoxin	*Liquid:* 0.05 mg/ml	**Loading dose:** *give ½ initially po/IM/IV, remaining*
(Lanoxin)	*Tab:* 0.125, 0.25, 0.5 mg	*in two equally divided doses Q 4h (IV) or Q 6-8h (po/IM).*
	Cap: 0.05, 0.1, 0.2 mg	**Maintenance:** give indicated dose QD.
	Inj: 0.1, 0.25 mg/ml	

	Loading		Maintenance	
	PO	IM/IV	PO	IM/IV
Premature	20 µg/kg	15	5 µg/kg	3.5
Full term	30	20	9	7
<2 y.o.	45	35	11	8.3
2-10 y.o.	35	25	9	7
>10 y.o.-adult	0.75-1.25 mg		0.125-0.25 mg	

Digitalis OD: see p. 130.

Digoxin immune FAB *(Digibind)*	*Inj:* 40 mg/4 ml	

Dihydroergotamine mesylate *(DHE-45)*	*Inj:* 1 mg/ml	**IM:** *Adult:* 1 mg Q 1h, max 3 doses/d. Max 6 mg/wk. **IV:** *Adult:* 1 mg Q 1h, max 2 doses/d. Max 6 mg/wk.

Diltiazem *(Cardizem, Dilacor XR)*	*Tab:* 30, 60, 90, 120 mg *Cap* (Cardizem SR): 60, 90, 120 mg *Cap* (Cardizem CD): 120, 180, 240, 300 mg *Cap* (Dilacor XR): 180, 240 mg *Inj:* 5 mg/ml	**PO:** *Adult: Angina:* 30-90 mg (tab) 4 times a day before meals and at hs or 120-480 mg QD (Cardizem CD). *Adult: HTN:* 60-120 mg po BID (Cardizem SR) or 180-240 mg po QD (Cardizem CD or Dilacor XR). **IV:** *Adult:* initial: 0.25 mg/kg IV over 2min. May repeat dose of 0.35 mg/kg if necessary. **Infusion:** *Adult:* start 5-10 mg/h after initial IV doses as above. May increase in 5 mg increments to max 15 mg/h for up to 24h.

Pediatric and Adult Drug Dosing

See index for generic names of proprietary meds

MEDICATION	PREPARATIONS	DOSING
Dimenhydrinate (*Dramamine, Dimetabs*)	*Liquid*: 12.5, 16 mg/ml *Tab (chew)/cap*: 50 mg *Inj*: 50 mg/ml	*Child 2-6 y.o.*: 1.25 mg/kg/dose po/IM Q 6h, max 75 mg/d. *Child 6-12 y.o.*: 1.25 mg/kg/dose po/IM Q 6h, max 150 mg/d. *Adult*: 50-100 mg po/IM/IV Q 4-6h, max 400 mg/d.
Diphenhydramine (*Benadryl*)	*Liquid*: 12.5 mg/5 ml *Tab/cap*: 25, 50 mg *Inj*: 50 mg/ml	*Child*: 1.25 mg/kg/dose po Q 6h. *Adult*: 25-50 mg po Q 6h.
Diphenoxylate/ atropine (*Lomotil*)	*Liquid*: Diphen 2.5 mg, atropine 0.025 mg/5 ml *Tab*: Diphen 2.5 mg, atropine 0.025 mg	*Child > 2 y.o.*: (as diphen.) 0.3-0.4 mg/kg/d po divided TID to QID. *Adult*: 1-2 tabs (or tsp) po TID to QID, decreasing as permitted by diarrhea to BID or TID.
Dipyridamole (*Persantine*)	*Tab*: 25, 50, 75 mg	*Adult*: 75-100 mg po QID.
Disopyramide (*Norpace*)	*Cap*: 100, 150 mg *Cap ext rel*: 100, 150 mg	*Child <1 y.o.*: 2.5-7.5 mg/kg/dose po Q 6h. *Child 1-4 y.o.*: 2.5-5.0 mg/kg/dose po Q 6h. *Child 4-12 y.o.*: 2.5-3.8 mg/kg/dose po Q 6h. *Child 12-18 y.o.*: 1.5-3.8 mg/kg/dose po Q 6h. *Adult*: 100-200 mg po Q 6h or (cap ext rel) 200-400 mg po Q 12h.
Disulfiram (*Antabuse*)	*Tab*: 250, 500 mg	*Adult*: 125-500 mg po Q AM.

Dobutamine (*Dobutrex*)	*Inj:* 250 mg/vial	*Child/adult:* 2-15 µg/kg/min, max 40 µg/kg/min. *See dosing table p. 152.*
Docusate sodium (*Colace*)	*Syrup:* 5, 20 mg/5 ml *Soln:* 50 mg/ml *Tab:* 50, 100 mg *Cap:* 50, 100, 240, 250, 300 mg	*Child <3 y.o.:* 10 mg/dose po QD-QID. *Child 3-6 y.o.:* 15 mg/dose po QD-QID. *Child 6-12 y.o.:* 40 mg/dose po QD-QID. *Child >12 y.o.-adult:* 50-125 mg/dose po QD-QID.
Dopamine (*Intropin, Dopastat*)	*Inj:* 40, 80, 160 mg/ml	*Child/adult:* 2-5 µg/kg/min IV= renal dose. 5-15 µg/kg/min IV = renal, ino- and chronotropic effects. >20 µg/kg/min IV = α adrenergic effects predominate. *See dosing table p. 153.*
Doxacurium chloride (*Nuromax*)	*Inj:* 1 mg/ml	*Child >2 y.o.:* 0.03 mg/kg IV, then 0.005-0.01 mg/kg prn. *Adult:* 0.05 mg/kg IV, then 0.005-0.01 mg/kg IV prn.
Doxazosin (*Cardura*)	*Tab:* 1, 2, 8 mg	*Adult:* 1-16 mg po QD.
Doxepin (*Sinequan, Adapin*)	*Liquid:* 10 mg/ml *Cap:* 10, 25, 50, 75, 100, 150 mg	*Adult:* 75-150 mg/d po in single or divided doses.
Doxycycline (*Vibramycin, Doxy-Caps, Doxychel*)	*Liquid:* 25, 50 mg/5 ml *Tab/cap:* 50, 100 mg *Inj:* 100, 200 mg	**PO:** *Child >8 y.o. and <45 kg:* 4.4 mg/kg/d on day 1 divided BID, then 2.2-4.4 mg/kg/d QD or divided BID. *Child >45 kg-adult:* 50-100 mg BID. **IV:** *Child >8 y.o. and <45 kg:* 4.4 mg/kg/d div Q 12h on day 1, then 2.2-4.4 mg/kg/d or div Q 12h. Max 200 mg/d. *Child >45 kg-adult:* 0.2 g/d QD or divided Q 12h on day 1, then 0.1-0.2 g/d QD or divided Q 12h. Max 300 mg/d.

Pediatric and Adult Drug Dosing

See index for generic names of proprietary meds

MEDICATION	PREPARATIONS	DOSING
Eflornithine (*Ornidyl*)	*Inj:* 200 mg/ml	***Pneumocystis pneumonia:*** *Adult:* 100 mg/kg/dose IV Q 6h over 45min for 14d.
Enalapril (*Vasotec*)	*Tab:* 2.5, 5, 10, 20 mg *Inj:* 1.25 mg/ml	**PO:** *Adult:* 5-40 mg/d QD or divided BID. **IV:** *Adult:* 1.25 mg Q 6h. Administer over 5min.
Enoxacin (*Penetrax*)	*Tab:* 200, 400 mg	*Adult >18 y.o.:* **UTI:** 400 mg po BID or 600 mg QD for 7-14d.
Epinephrine	*Inj:* 1:10,000 (1 mg/10 ml), 1:1,000 (1 mg/1 ml)	**CPR/VF:** *Child:* 0.1 ml (1:10,000)/kg/dose IV/ET Q 5min. *Adult:* 10 ml = 1 mg (1:10,000) IV / ET Q 5min. **Anaphylaxis:** *Child:* 0.1 ml (1:10,000)/kg/dose (max 5 ml) IV over 5min. *Adult:* 1.0-5.0 ml (1:10,000) IV over 5min. **Asthma:** *Child:* 0.01 ml (1:1,000)/kg/dose (max 0.3 ml) SC Q 20min prn x 3. *Adult:* 0.3 ml (1:1,000) SC Q 20min prn x 3.
Epinephrine, racemic	*Sltn:* 22.5 mg/ml (7.5, 15, 30 ml)	*Child/adult:* 0.05 ml/kg/dose (*child*) or 0.5 ml (*adult*) with 2 ml NS over 15min nebulized. Repeat Q 2h as needed.
Ergotamine (*Ergomar, Ergostat, Medihaler-Ergotamine*)	*Subling tab:* 2 mg Aerosol inhaler: 360 μg/metered spray	**SL:** *Child 12-18 y.o.:* 1 mg Q 30min, max 3 mg/d. *Adult:* 2 mg, then 1-2 mg Q 30min, max 6 mg/d or 10 mg/wk.

		Inhaled: 1 metered inhalation. If headache not relieved, repeat Q 5min to max 6 inhalations/d or 15/wk.
Ergotamine/caffeine (*Cafergot*)	*Tab:* Ergot 1 mg, caffeine 100 mg *Supp:* Ergot 2 mg, caffeine 100 mg	*Adult:* 2 tabs po, then 1 tab po Q 30min, max 6 tabs/d or 1 supp PR, then 2nd supp 1h later if needed, max 2 supp/attack.
Erythromycin base (*E-mycin, Eryc, Ethril 500, Eryped Erythrocin, Robimycin*)	*Tab:* 250, 500 mg *Tab (enteric coated):* 250, 330, 500 mg *Pellets (enteric coated):* 125, 250 mg	**PO:** *Child:* 7.5-12.5 mg/kg/dose (max 500 mg/dose) Q 6h. *Adult:* 250-500 mg Q 6h.
Erythromycin estolate (*Ilosone*)	*Drops:* 100 mg/ml *Susp:* 125, 250 mg/5 ml *Tab:* 250, 500 mg *Tab (chew):* 125, 250 mg *Cap:* 125, 250 mg	**PO:** *Child:* 7.5-12.5 mg/kg/dose (max 500 mg/dose) Q 6h. *Adult:* 250-500 mg Q 6h. Avoid treatment for longer than 10d or for repeated courses to decrease likelihood of hepatotoxicity.
Erythromycin ethylsuccinate (*E.E.S.*)	*Liquid:* 200, 400 mg/5ml *Granules for oral susp (as liquid):* 400 mg/5ml *Drops:* 100 mg/2.5 ml *Tab:* 200, 400 mg	**PO:** *Child:* 7.5-12.5 mg/kg/dose (max 500 mg/dose) Q 6h. *Adult:* 400-800 mg Q 6h.
Erythromycin lacto-bionate or gluceptate	*Inj:* 0.5, 1.0 g	**IV:** *Child:* 5.0-12.5 mg/kg/dose Q 6h. *Adult:* 0.5-1 g Q 6h.

Pediatric and Adult Drug Dosing

See index for generic names of proprietary meds

MEDICATION	PREPARATIONS	DOSING
Erythromycin stearate *(Erythrocin stearate, Erypar filmseal, Ethril, Wyamycin S)*	*Tab:* 250, 500 mg	**PO:** *Child:* 7.5-12.5 mg/kg/dose (max 500 mg) Q 6h. *Adult:* 250-500 mg Q 6h.
Erythromycin/ sulfisoxazole *(Pediazole)*	*Susp:* Erythro 200 mg, Sulf 600 mg/5 ml	*Child >2 mo.:* 0.3 ml/kg/dose po Q 6h, max 6 g sulfisoxazole/d.
Esmolol *(Brevibloc)*	*Inj:* 100 mg/vial; 2.5g/ampule	*Child/adult:* 500 µg/kg loading dose over 1min IV, then 50 µg/kg/min infusion. If no effect in 4min, repeat loading dose and increase infusion to 100 µg/kg/min. May repeat loading dose in 4min and increase infusion by 50 µg/kg/min two additional times, to max infusion rate of 200 µg/kg/min. *See dosing table p.* 154.
Ethambutol *(Myambutol)*	*Tab:* 100, 400 mg	*Child: >13 y.o.-adult:* **TB initial Rx:** 15 mg/kg/dose po QD. **Re-Rx:** 25 mg/kg/dose po QD for 60d, then 15 mg/kg QD.
Ethionamide *(Trecator-SC)*	*Tab:* 250 mg	*Adult:* 500-1000 mg/d po divided QD-TID.
Ethosuximide *(Zarontin)*	*Liquid:* 250 mg/5 ml *Cap:* 250 mg	**Seizure maintenance:** *Child >3 y.o.:* 20-30 mg/kg/d po divided BID, max 1500 mg/d. *Adult:* 250-1500 mg/d po divided BID.

Drug	Forms	Dosage
Etodolac (*Lodine*)	*Cap:* 200, 300 mg *Tab:* 400 mg	*Adult:* **Pain:** 200-400 mg po TID-QID prn. **DJD:** 600-1200 mg/d as 200 mg po TID-QID, 300 mg po BID-QID, or 400 mg po BID-TID. *Max 1200 mg/d; if < 60 kg, 20 mg/kg/d.*
Famciclovir (*Famvir*)	*Tab:* 500 mg	**Herpes zoster:** *Adult:* 500 mg po Q 8h for 7d.
Famotidine (*Pepcid*)	*Liquid:* 40 mg/5 ml *Tab:* 20, 40 mg *Inj:* 10 mg/ml	**PO:** *Child:* 1.0-1.2 mg/kg/d divided Q 8-12h, max 40 mg/d. *Adult:* 20-80 mg/d divided Q 12-24h. **IV:** *Child:* 0.6-0.8 mg/kg/d divided Q 8-12h, max 40 mg/d. *Adult:* 20 mg Q 12h.
Felodipine (*Plendil*)	*Tab:* 5, 10 mg	*Adult:* usual 5-10 mg po QD, max 20 mg po QD.
Fenoprofen (*Nalfon*)	*Tab:* 600 mg *Cap:* 200, 300 mg	*Adult:* **Pain:** 200 po mg Q 4-6h prn. **Arthritis:** 300-600 mg TID-QID, max 3.2 g/d.
Fentanyl (*Sublimaze*)	*Inj:* 50 μg/ml	*Child:* 2 μg/kg IV over 3min Q 30min prn. *Adult:* 50-100 μg over 3min Q 30min prn.
Ferrous fumarate (33% elemental iron) (*Femiron, Feostat, Fumasorb, Fumerin, Hemocyte, Ircon-FA*)	*Susp:* 100 mg/5 ml; 45 mg/0.6 ml *Tab:* 63, 195, 200, 325 mg *Tab (chew):* 100 mg *Tab (ext rel):* 325 mg	**Iron deficiency anemia:** *Adult:* 200 mg po TID or QID. *Ext rel tab:* 325 mg po BID.

Pediatric and Adult Drug Dosing

See index for generic names of proprietary meds

MEDICATION	PREPARATIONS	DOSING
Ferrous gluconate (12% elemental iron) (*Fergon, Ferralet, Simron*)	*Liquid:* 300 mg/5 ml *Tab:* 300, 320, 325 mg *Cap:* 86, 325 mg	**Iron deficiency anemia:** *Child >2 y.o.:* 8-16 mg/kg/dose po Q 8h. *Adult:* 325 mg po Q 8h.
Ferrous sulfate (20% elemental iron) (*Feosol, Fer-IN-Sol, Fer-Iron, Fero-Gradumet, Ferospace, Ferralyn, Ferra-TD, Mol-Iron, Slow Fe*)	*Elixir:* 220 mg/5 ml *Syrup:* 90 mg/5 ml *Tab:* 160, 195, 300, 325 mg *Cap:* 150, 190, 250, 390 mg	**Iron deficiency anemia:** *Child >2 y.o.:* 5-10 mg/kg/dose po Q 8h. *Adult:* 300 mg/dose po Q 8h.
Finasteride (*Proscar*)	*Tab:* 5 mg	**BPH:** 5 mg po QD.
Flavoxate (*Urispas*)	*Tab:* 100 mg	*Child >12 y.o.-adult:* 100-200 mg po Q 6-8h.
Flecainide (*Tambocor*)	*Tab:* 50, 100, 150 mg	*Adult:* 50-200 mg po Q 12h.

Fluconazole *(Diflucan)*	*Tab:* 50, 100, 150, 200 mg *Inj:* 2 mg/ml	*Child 3-13 y.o.:* ***All indications:*** initial dose 10 mg/kg po/IV, then 3-6 mg/kg/dose po/IV QD. *Child >13 y.o.-adult:* ***Oral/esophageal candidiasis:*** start 200 mg po/IV on day 1, then 100 mg po/IV QD. Up to 400 mg/d has been used. ***Candida/yeast*** ***vaginitis:*** 150 mg po single dose. ***Systemic candidiasis:*** 400 mg po/IV on day 1, then 200 mg po/IV QD. ***Cryptococcal meningitis:*** 400 mg po/IV on day 1, then 200 mg po/IV QD. Up to 400 mg/d has been used.
Flucytosine *(Ancobon)*	*Liquid:* 10 mg/ml (prepared by pharmacist) *Cap:* 250, 500 mg	*PO: Child <50 kg:* 1.5-4.5 g/m²/d divided Q 6h. *Child >50 kg-adult:* 50-150 mg/kg/d divided Q 6h. See p. 165 for body surface area determination.
Flumazenil *(Mazicon,* *Romazicon)*	*Inj:* 0.1 mg/ml (5, 10 ml)	***Reversal of sedative effect of benzodiazepines given by medical*** ***personnel:*** *Child/adult:* 0.2 mg IV over 15sec. If no effect 45sec later, repeat same dose. May repeat at 1min intervals until total 1 mg given. ***Suspected benzodiazepine OD:*** *Child/adult:* 0.2 mg IV over 30sec. If no effect, try 0.3 mg IV over 30sec. If still no effect, try 0.5 mg IV over 30sec, then repeat Q 1min until total 3 mg given.
Flunisolide *(Aerobid)*	*Inhaler:* 250 µg/puff *Nasal spray:* 25 µg/spray	**Inhaler:** *Child 6-15 y.o.:* 2 puffs BID. *Child >15 y.o.-adult:* 2-4 puffs BID. **Nasal spray:** *Child 6-15 y.o.-adult:* 2 sprays per nostril BID. *Child >15 y.o.-adult:* 2 sprays per nostril BID-QID.

Pediatric and Adult Drug Dosing

See index for generic names of proprietary meds

MEDICATION	PREPARATIONS	DOSING
Fluoxetine (*Prozac*)	*Liquid:* 20 mg/5 ml *Cap:* 10, 20 mg	*Adult:* 20-80 po mg/d. Start at 20 mg po Q AM. For larger doses give two times a day with second dose at noon.
Fluphenazine (*Prolixin*)	*Liquid:* 2.5 mg/5 ml; 5 mg/ml *Tab:* 1, 2.5, 5, 10 mg *Inj:* 2.5 mg/ml Long acting inj: 25 mg/ml	**PO:** *Adult:* 2.5-10 mg/d divided TID-QID, max 20 mg/d. **IM:** *Adult:* 1.25-10 mg Q 6-8h. **LA Inj:** *Adult:* 12.5-25 mg IM Q 2wk.
Flurbiprofen (*Ansaid*)	*Tab:* 50, 100 mg	*Adult:* 200-300 mg/d po, divided BID, TID, or QID.
Folic acid	*Tab:* 0.1, 0.4, 0.8, 1.0 mg	**Folic acid deficiency:** *Child <4 y.o.:* 0.3 mg QD. *Child >4 y.o.-adult:* 1 mg QD.
Fosinopril (*Monopril*)	*Tab:* 10, 20 mg	*Adult:* start 10 mg po QD, adjust by response, usual dose 20-40 mg, max 80 mg/d in single or divided doses.
Furazolidone (*Furoxone*)	*Liquid:* 50 mg/15 ml *Tab:* 100 mg	**Giardiasis:** see p. 13.
Furosemide (*Lasix*)	*Liquid:* 10 mg/ml, 40 mg/5 ml *Tab:* 20, 40, 80 mg *Inj:* 10 mg/ml	**PO:** *Child:* initial 2 mg/kg/dose Q 6-8h. *Adult:* start 20-80 mg Q 12-24h. **IV:** *Child:* 1 mg/kg/dose. *Adult:* 40-60 mg/dose as initial Rx of CHF; double dose if

		no diuresis in 30min. Adjust dose upward for renal insufficiency or failure.
Gabapentin (*Neurontin*)	*Cap:* 100, 300, 400 mg	*Child >12 y.o.-adult:* 300-600 mg/dose po TID.
Ganciclovir (*Cytovene*)	*Inj:* 500 mg	*Child >12 y.o.-adult:* 5 mg/kg/dose Q 12h IV for 14-21d, then 5 mg/kg/dose IV QD.
Gemfibrozil (*Lopid*)	*Tab:* 600 mg *Cap:* 300 mg	*Adult:* 600 mg po 30min before morning and evening meals.
Gentamicin (*Garamycin*)	*Inj:* 40 mg/ml (adult); 10 mg/ml (pediatric); 2 mg/ml (intrathecal)	*Child <7 days:* 2.5 mg/kg/dose IM/IV Q12h. *Child >7 days:* 2.5 mg/kg/dose IM/IV Q 8h, max 300 mg/d. *Adult:* load 2 mg IM/IV, then 1.7 mg/kg Q 8h IM/IV. Alternate QD dosing (adult only): 5.1 mg/kg IM/IV.
Glipizide (*Glucotrol*)	*Tab:* 5, 10 mg	*Adult:* 2.5-40 mg/d po QD or divided BID.
Glucagon	*Inj:* 1 mg/ml	***Calcium channel blocker or β- blocker OD:*** *Child:* 50 μg/kg IV over 5min. *Adult:* 5-10 mg IV over 1min. *See also p.128.*
Glyburide (*Micronase, DiaBeta, Glynase*)	*Tab:* 1.25, 2.5, 5 mg <u>Glynase PresTab</u>: 1.5, 3 mg	*Adult (tab):* 1.25-20 mg po QD. *Adult* (<u>Glynase PresTab</u>): 0.75-12 mg po QD. *Regular tab 5 mg equivalent in potency to PresTab 3 mg.*
Glycerin (*Osmoglyn*)	*Oral soltn:* 0.628 g/ml (50%)	*Adult:* 1.0-1.8 g/kg po Q5h. Give in chilled solution mixed with lemon juice.

Pediatric and Adult Drug Dosing

See index for generic names of proprietary meds

MEDICATION	PREPARATIONS	DOSING
Glycopyrrolate (*Robinul*)	*Tab:* 1, 2 mg *Inj:* 0.2 mg/ml	**PO:** *Child > 12 y.o.-adult:* 1-2 mg/dose BID-QID. **IV: Reversal of NM blockade:** *Child/adult:* 0.2 mg per mg of neostigmine being administered simultaneously.
Griseofulvin (*Fulvicin, Grisactin, Grifulvin*)	**Microsize:** *Tab:* 250, 500 mg *Cap:* 125, 250 mg *Liquid:* 125 mg/5 ml **Ultramicrosize:** *Tab:* 125, 165, 250, 330 mg	**Microsize:** *Child > 2 y.o.:* 10-20 mg/kg/dose po QD. *Adult:* 500-1000 mg/d po QD or divided BID. **Ultramicrosize:** *Child > 2 y.o.:* 7 mg/kg/d po divided BID. *Adult:* 330-750 mg/d po QD or divided BID. *Give with fatty foods to avoid GI distress.*
Guanabenz (*Wytensin*)	*Tab:* 4, 8 mg	*Child 12-18 y.o.:* 0.04-0.1 mg/kg/dose po BID. *Adult:* 4-32 mg po Q12h.
Guanfacine (*Tenex*)	*Tab:* 1, 2 mg	*Adult:* 1-2 mg po Qhs.
Haloperidol (*Haldol*)	*Liquid:* 2 mg/ml *Tab:* 0.5, 1, 2, 5, 10, 20 mg *Inj:* 5 mg/ml	**PO:** *Child 3-12 y.o.:* 0.01-0.03 mg/kg/dose QD-TID. *Child > 12 y.o.-adult:* 2-5 mg BID-TID. **IM:** *Child > 12 y.o.-adult:* 2-5 mg Q1h as needed.
Heparin	*Inj:* 10, 100, 1000, 2500, 5000, 7500, 10000, 20000, 40000 units/ml	**Myocardial infarction:** see p. 20. **Pulmonary embolus:** see p. 27. **Venous thrombosis, deep:** see p. 34.
Hepatitis B immune globulin (*Hep-B-Gammagee, Hyper-Hep, H-BIG*)	*Inj:* 0.5, 1, 5 ml	*Neonates born of HBsAg-positive mothers:* 0.5 ml IM at birth. *Child > 1 mo.-adult:* 0.06 ml/kg IM. *Also give Hepatitis B vaccine—* see p. 15, 67.

Drug	Forms	Dosing
Hepatitis B vaccine (Recombivax HB, Engerix-B)	Recombivax HB: 1.25, 5, 10, 15, 30, 40 µg/vial Engerix-B: 10, 20 µg/vial	Post-exposure give Hep. B imm. globulin also—see p. 15, 66. For *pediatric vaccination schedule* see p. 175. Give IM in indicated doses at 0, 1, and 6 months.

	Recombivax HB	Engerix-B
Infants of HBsAg-neg mothers and child <11 y.o.	2.5 µg	10 µg
Infants of HBsAg-pos mothers	5 µg	10 µg
Child 11-19 y.o.	5 µg	20 µg
Adults >19 y.o.	10 µg	20 µg
Dialysis/immunocompromised adults	40 µg	40 µg

Drug	Forms	Dosing
Hydralazine (Apresoline)	Tab: 10, 25, 50, 100 mg Inj: 20 mg/ml	PO: *Child:* 0.2-1.8 mg/kg/dose Q 6h, max 25 mg/dose. *Adult:* 10-100 mg Q 6h. IM/IV: *Child:* 0.1-0.2 mg/kg/dose Q 4-6h, max 20 mg/dose. *Adult:* 5-20 mg IV Q 20min prn; 10-50 mg IM Q 3-6h prn.
Hydrochlorothiazide (Esidrix, Hydrodiuril)	Liquid: 50 mg/5 ml Tab: 25, 50, 100 mg	*Child:* 1.0-1.5 mg/kg/dose po BID. *Adult:* 25-100 mg/d po QD or divided BID.
Hydrochlorothiazide/ spironolactone (Aldactazide)	Tab: Hydro 25 mg, Spiro 25 mg; Hydro 50 mg, Spiro 50 mg	*Child:* as spironolact 1.65-3.3 mg/kg/d po QD or divided BID. *Adult:* as spironolact 25-100 mg/dose po QD-BID.
Hydrochlorothiazide/ triamterene (Dyazide, Maxzide)	Cap: Hydro 25 mg, Triam 37.5 mg; Hydro 50 mg, Triam 37.5 mg	*Adult:* 1-2 caps po QD.

Pediatric and Adult Drug Dosing

See index for generic names of proprietary meds

MEDICATION	PREPARATIONS	DOSING
Hydrocodone/ acetaminophen (*Vicodin, Vicodin ES*)	*Liquid:* Hy 2.5 mg, Acet 120 mg/5 ml *Tab:* Hy 2.5 or 7.5 mg, Acet 500 mg; Hy 5 mg, Acet 500 mg; Hy 7.5 mg, Acet 750 mg; Hy 7.5 or 10 mg, Acet 650 mg	*Child:* as hydrocodone 0.125 mg/kg/dose po QID. *Adult:* as hydrocodone 5-10 mg po Q 4-6h.
Hydrocortisone (*Solu-Cortef*)	*Liquid:* 10 mg/5 ml *Tab:* 5, 10, 20 mg *Inj:* 100, 250, 500, 1000 mg/vial	*Dosage dependent on disease process undergoing treatment.*
Ibuprofen (*Motrin, Advil, Nuprin*)	*Liquid:* 100 mg/5 ml *Tab:* 200, 300, 400, 600, 800 mg	*Child >12 mo.:* 5-10 mg/kg/dose po Q 6-8h. *Adult:* 200-800 mg po Q 6-8h.
Imipenem/cilastatin (*Primaxin*)	*Inj:* 250, 500 mg	*Child >11 y.o.:* 12.5 mg/kg/dose IV Q 6h, max 4 g/d. *Adult:* 0.5-1.0 g IV Q 6h.
Imipramine (*Tofranil*)	*Tab:* 10, 25, 50 mg	***Enuresis:*** *Child >6 y.o.:* 25-75 mg po 1h before hs, max if <12 y.o. 50 mg. ***Depression:*** *Adult:* 100-300 mg po divided BID-TID.
Indapamide (*Lozol*)	*Tab:* 1.25, 2.5 mg	*Adult:* 2.5-5 mg po QD.

Indomethacin *(Indocin)*	*Liquid:* 25 mg/5 ml *Cap:* 25, 50 mg *Cap (SR):* 75 mg *Supp:* 50 mg	***Gout attack, acute:*** p. 14. *Other:* 75-200 mg/d po or PR divided TID-QID.
Ipratropium bromide *(Atrovent)*	*Inhaler:* 18 µg/puff *Inhalation sltn:* 500 µg/vial	**Inhaler:** *Adult:* 1-2 puffs TID-QID. May be taken more frequently as needed, not to exceed 12 inhalations/24h. **Nebulized:** *Adult:* 500 µg in 2.5 ml NS Q 6-8h.
Isoetharine *(Bronkosol)*	*Inhaler:* 340 µg/puff *Inhalation solution:* mult concentrations	**Inhaler:** *Adult:* 1-2 puffs Q 3-4h. **Nebulized:** *Child:* 0.1-0.2 mg/kg/dose with 2 ml NS Q2-6h. *Adult:* 5 mg with 2 ml NS nebulized Q2-6h.
Isoniazid *(INH)*	*Tab:* 50, 100, 300 mg *Oral solution:* 50 mg/5 ml	*Child:* 10 mg/kg/dose (max 300 mg) po QD. *Adult:* 300 mg po QD.
Isoproterenol *(Isuprel)*	*Inhaler:* 120, 131 µg/puff *Inhalation sltn:* 0.25%, 0.5%, 1% *Inj:* 200 µg/ml	**Inhaler:** *Child/adult:* 1-2 puffs Q 4h prn. **Nebulized:** *Child:* 0.05 mg/kg/dose (min 0.5 mg, max 1.25 mg) diluted with 2 ml NS Q4h. *Adult:* 2.5-5.0 mg dilute with 2 ml NS Q4h. **IV:** *Heart block: Child:* start 0.1 µg/kg/min, titrate to max 1.5 µg/kg/min infusion. *Adult:* start 2 µg/min, titrate to max 10 µg/min infusion.

Pediatric and Adult Drug Dosing

See index for generic names of proprietary meds

MEDICATION	PREPARATIONS	DOSING
Isosorbide dinitrate *(Isordil, Sorbitrate)*	*Subling tab:* 2.5, 5, 10 mg *Tab (chew):* 5, 10 mg (Sorbitrate) *Tab:* 5, 10, 20, 30, 40 mg *Tab (LA):* 40 mg (scored) (Isordil, Dilatrate SR)	**Sublingual or chew tab:** 2.5-10 mg Q 5min prn pain or before activity likely to cause angina. **Tab:** 5-40 mg po Q 6-8h. **LA tab:** 20-40 mg Q 6-12h or 80 mg Q 8-12h. *Use smallest effective dose.*
Isradipine *(DynaCirc)*	*Tab:* 2.5, 5 mg	*Adult:* 2.5-10 mg po BID.
Itraconazole *(Sporanox)*	*Caps:* 100 mg	*Adult:* 200 mg po QD with food. Increase in 100 mg increments to max 400 mg/d. If giving more than 200 mg/d, divide BID.
Kayexalate	*Liquid:* 15 g/60 ml *Powder:* 3.5 g/5 ml	*Child:* 1 g/kg/dose po or as retention enema Q 2-6h. *Adult:* 15-60 g po or 30-50 g as retention enema Q 2-6h.
Ketamine *(Ketalar)*	*Inj:* 10, 50, 100 mg/ml	***Sedation for rapid sequence intubation:*** *Child/adult:* 2-5 mg/kg rapidly IV. See p. 150-151 for RSI protocol.
Ketoconazole *(Nizoral)*	*Liquid:* 100 mg/5 ml *Tab:* 200 mg *Cream:* 2%	*Dosage dependent on disease process undergoing treatment.*

Ketoprofen (*Orudis*)	*Tab:* 25, 50, 75 mg	*Adult:* 25-75 mg TID-QID.
Ketorolac (*Toradol*)	*Tab:* 10 mg *Inj:* 15, 30 mg/ml	*Should only be used short term—adverse effects are common.* **PO:** *Adult:* 10 mg Q4-6h, max 40 mg/d. **IM:** *Adult:* start 60 mg, then ½ initial dose Q6h prn, max 120 mg/d. *Adult > 65 y.o.:* halve doses.
Labetalol (*Trandate, Normodyne*)	*Tab:* 100, 200, 300 mg *Inj:* 5 mg/ml (20, 40 ml)	**PO:** *Adult:* usual 100-400 mg Q12h. Max 2.4 g/d div TID. **IV:** *Adult:* 20 mg over 2min, then 40-80 mg Q10min, max total 300 mg. **IV infusion for hypertensive emergency:** *Adult:* start 2 mg/min, titrate. Max total 300 mg.
Lactulose (*Cephulac*)	*Liquid:* 10 g/15 ml	**Constipation:** *Adult:* 15-30 ml po QID. **Hepatic encephalopathy:** *Adult:* 30-45 ml po TID-QID or 300 ml diluted with 700 ml NS as retention enema Q4-6h.
Laudanum		See p. 84.
Levodopa (*L-Dopa*)	*Tab:* 100, 250, 500 mg *Cap:* 100, 250, 500 mg	*Adult:* start 0.5-1.0 g/d, divided BID, TID, or QID with food May increase by up to 0.75 g/d Q3-7d. Usual maintenance 3-6 g/d, divided TID. Max 8 g/d. Usually given in combination with carbidopa as <u>Sinemet</u>—see below.
Levodopa/carbidopa (*Sinemet*)	*Tab:* Lev 100 mg, carb 10 mg (<u>Sinemet 10-100</u>); Lev 100 mg, carb 25 mg (<u>Sinemet 25-100</u>); Lev 250 mg, carb 25 mg (<u>Sinemet 25-250</u>)	*Adult:* usual starting dose 1 tab <u>Sinemet 25-100</u> TID. Dose may be increased by 1 tab <u>Sinemet 25-100</u> every 1-2d to obtain desired effect. Usual maintenance 1-2 tabs <u>Sinemet</u> <u>25-250</u> TID. Dose range of carbidopa usually 70-200 mg/d.

Pediatric and Adult Drug Dosing

MEDICATION	PREPARATIONS	DOSING
Levothyroxine (*Synthroid, Levothroid, Levoxine*)	*Tab:* 25, 50, 75, 87, 100, 112, 125, 150, 175, 200, 300 µg *Inj:* 200, 500 µg	**Maintenance:** *Child <6 mo.:* 25-50 µg or 8-10 µg/kg po QD. *Child 6-12 mo.:* 50-75 µg or 6-8 µg/kg QD. *Child 1-5 y.o.:* 75-100 µg or 5-6 µg/kg QD. *Child 6-12 y.o.:* 100-150 µg or 4-5 µg/kg QD. *Child >12 y.o.:* 150 µg or 2-3 µg/kg QD. *Adult:* 100-200 µg (= 0.1-0.2 mg) QD. **New dx hypothyroidism:** start 50 µg/d, may increase by 25-50 µg/d Q 2-4wk until desired effect obtained. **Hypothyroid coma:** see p. 16.
Lidocaine (*Xylocaine*)	*Inj:* 10, 20, 40, 200 mg/ml *Viscous oral susp:* 2 g/100 ml	**VF/VT:** *Child:* 1 mg/kg/dose IV. May repeat in 10-15min, then start 20-50 µg/kg/min infusion. *Adult:* 50-100 mg (or 1 mg/kg) IV, then 2-4 mg/min infusion. Repeat bolus 50-75 mg (or 0.5 mg/kg) IV as necessary 5-10min, max total of boluses 225 mg. *Reduce dose by 50% for CHF, shock, or if age >70 y.o.* **Oral topical anesthesia:** *Child/adult:* 15 ml swished around mouth and spit out or swallow Q 3-8h as needed.
Lindane (Gamma benzene hexachloride) (*Kwell*)	*Lotion, cream, shampoo:* 1%	**Lice:** see p. 28. **Scabies:** see p. 28.
Liothyronine (*Cytomel*)	*Tab:* 5, 25, 50 µg	*Adult:* usual maintenance 25-75 µg po QD. To initiate Rx, start 25 µg QD. May increase by 12.5-25 µg/dose Q 1-2wk.

Lisinopril *(Prinivil, Zestril)*	*Tab:* 5, 10, 20, 40 mg	*Adult:* 10-80 mg po QD.
Lithium *(Eskalith, Cibalith, Lithobid, Lithotab Lithonate)*	*Liquid:* 300 mg/5 ml *Tab/Cap:* 150, 300, 600 mg *Tab (SR):* 300 (Lithobid), 450 mg (Eskalith CR)	***Maintenance:*** *Child:* 15-60 mg/kg/d po. *Adult:* 900-1200 mg/d po. Divide as follows: Liquid and tab/cap: TID-QID; Eskalith CR: BID; Lithobid: BID-TID.
Lomefloxacin *(Maxaquin)*	*Tab:* 400 mg	*Adult: UTI, lower resp infection:* 400 mg po QD for 7-14d.
Loperamide *(Imodium)*	*Liquid:* 1 mg/5 ml *Cap:* 2 mg *Tab:* 2 mg	*Child 2-5 y.o.:* 1 mg po TID on day 1. *Child 6-8 y.o.:* 2 mg po BID on day 1. *Child 9-12 y.o.:* 2 mg po TID on day 1. *Child >12 y.o.-adult:* start 4 mg po, then give 2 mg po after each unformed stool. Max 16 mg/d. *Maintenance dose on day 2 is ¹/₃ to ¹/₂ of initial dose.*
Loracarbef *(2nd gen)* *(Lorabid)*	*Liquid:* 100 mg/5 ml *Cap:* 200 mg	*PO: Child >6 mo.: Acute OM:* 15 mg/kg/dose Q 12h for 10d. **Other:** 7.5 mg/kg/dose Q 12h for 7-10d. *Adult: Resp/skin infections:* 200-400 mg Q 12h for 14d. *Lower UTI:* 200 mg QD for 7d. *Pyelo:* 400 mg BID for 14d.
Lorazepam *(Ativan)*	*Liquid:* 2, 4 mg/ml *Tab:* 0.5, 1, 2 mg *Inj:* 2, 4 mg/ml	*PO: Child:* 0.05 mg/kg/dose Q8h. *Adult:* 1-10 mg/d divided BID-TID. *IV: Sedation: Child:* 0.05 mg/kg/dose (max 4 mg). *Adult:* 2-4 mg/dose. *Alcohol withdrawal:* see p. 6.

Pediatric and Adult Drug Dosing

See index for generic names of proprietary meds

MEDICATION	PREPARATIONS	DOSING
Lovastatin (Mevacor)	Tab: 20, 40 mg	*Adult:* start 20 mg po with dinner. For extremely high cholesterol, may start at 40 mg/d. Increase dose Q 4wk until desired effect. Max 80 mg/d in single or div doses.
Loxapine (Loxitane)	Liquid: 25 mg/ml Tab: 5, 10, 25, 50 mg Inj: 50 mg/ml	**PO:** *Adult:* 10-50 mg/dose BID. **IM:** *Adult:* 12.5-50 mg Q 4-6h prn.
Magnesium citrate	Liquid: 16.17% (300 ml)	*Child 2-5 y.o.:* 25-75 ml po QD. *Child 6-11 y.o.:* 50-150 ml po QD. *Child >12 y.o.-adult:* 100-300 ml po QD.
Magnesium sulfate	Inj: 100, 125, 250, 500 mg/ml (0.8, 1, 2, 4 mEq/ml)	**IV:** *Child/adult:* 25-50 mg (0.2-0.4 mEq)/kg/dose Q 4-6h. Larger doses may be needed for severe hypomagnesemia. **Eclampsia:** see p. 9.
Mannitol (Osmitrol)	Inj: 50, 100, 150, 200, 250 mg/ml	**Increased intracranial pressure:** *Child/adult:* initial dose 0.25-2.0 g/kg IV, then 0.25 g/kg/dose IV as needed.
Maprotiline (Ludiomil)	Tab: 25, 50, 75 mg	*Adult:* 25-150 po QD or in divided doses. In some severely depressed patients, up to 225 mg/d may be given.
Mebendazole (Vermox)	Tab (chew): 100 mg	**Worms:** see p. 35.
Meclizine (Antivert)	Tab: 12.5, 25, 50 mg Tab (chew): 25 mg	**Vertigo:** *Child >12 y.o.-adult:* 25-100 mg/d divided Q 6-12h.

Meclofenamate *(Meclomen)*	*Cap:* 50, 100 mg	*Child >14 y.o.-adult:* 50-100 mg po Q 6-8h.
Mefenamic acid *(Ponstel)*	*Cap:* 250 mg	*Child >14 y.o.-adult:* 500 mg po, then 250 mg po Q 6h for up to 1 week.
Meperidine *(Demerol)*	*Liquid:* 50 mg/5 ml *Tab:* 50, 100 mg *Inj:* 25, 50, 75, 100 mg/ml	**PO/SC/IM/IV:** *Child:* 1.0-1.5 mg/kg/dose Q3-4h, max 100 mg/dose. *Adult:* 50-150 mg Q 3-4h prn.
Metaproterenol *(Alupent)*	*Liquid:* 10 mg/5 ml *Tab:* 10, 20 mg *Inhaler:* 650 µg/puff *Inhalation sltn:* 0.4, 0.6, 5%	**PO:** *Child < 6 y.o:* 0.3-0.6 mg/kg/dose Q 4-6h. *Child 6-9 y.o:* 10 mg Q 6-8h. *Adult:* 20 mg Q 6-8h. **Inhaler:** *Child/adult:* 1-3 puffs Q 3-4h, max 12 puffs/d. **Nebulized:** *Child:* 5-15 mg (0.1-0.3 ml of 5%) in 2.5 ml NS Q 4-6h. *Adult:* 15 mg (0.3 ml of 5%) in 2.5 ml NS Q 4-6h.
Methadone *(Dolophine)*	*Liquid:* 5, 10 mg/5 ml *Tab:* 5, 10 mg *Inj:* 10 mg/ml	**PO:** *Adult:* 5-20 mg Q 6-8h. **SC/IM/IV:** *Adult:* 2.5-10 mg Q 3-4h prn.
Methazolamide *(Neptazane)*	*Tab:* 25, 50 mg	*Adult:* 50-100 mg po BID-TID.
Methenamine hippurate *(Hiprex, Urex)*	*Tab:* 1 g (scored)	*Child 6-12 y.o.:* 0.5-1.0 g po Q12h. *Child >12 y.o.-adult:* 1.0 g po Q12h.
Methenamine mandelate *(Mandelamine)*	*Liquid:* 200, 500 mg/5 ml *Tab:* 500, 1000 mg	*Child <6 y.o.:* 50 mg/kg/d po divided after meals and at hs. *Child 6-12 y.o.:* 500 mg po QID. *Child 12 y.o.-adult:* 1 g po QID.

Pediatric and Adult Drug Dosing

See index for generic names of proprietary meds

MEDICATION	PREPARATIONS	DOSING
Methenamine/ phenylsalicylate/ atropine/ hyoscyamine (*Urised*)	*Tab*: Meth 40.8 mg, Phen 18.1 mg, Atro 0.03 mg, Hyos 0.03 mg	*Adult*: 2 tabs po Q 6h.
Methicillin (*Staphcillin*)	*Inj*: 1, 4, 6 g	**IM/IV**: *Child > 1 mo.*: 100-400 mg/kg/d divided Q 4-6h. *Adult*: 1-2 g Q 4h.
Methimazole (*Tapazole*)	*Tab*: 5, 10 mg	*Child*: 0.13 mg/kg/dose Q 8h po until hyperthyroidism controlled, then 0.067 mg/kg/dose po Q 8h. *Adult*: 5-20 mg Q 8h po until hyperthyroidism controlled, then 5-10 mg po Q 8-24h.
Methocarbamol (*Robaxin*)	*Tab*: 500, 750 mg *Inj*: 100 mg/ml	**PO**: *Adult*: 1500-2000 mg Q 6h. **IM/IV**: *Adult*: 1000 mg Q 8h. Max IM: 500 mg/site.
Methsuximide (*Celontin*)	*Cap*: 150, 300 mg	*Child*: 2.5-7.5 mg/kg/dose po Q 6h. *Adult*: 150-300 mg po Q 6-12h.
Methyclothiazide (*Enduron*)	*Tab*: 2.5, 5 mg	*Child*: 0.05-0.2 mg/kg/dose po QD. *Adult*: 2.5-10 mg po QD.
Methyldopa (*Aldomet*)	*Liquid*: 250 mg/5 ml *Tab*: 125, 250, 500 mg	**PO**: *Child*: 2.5-16.25 mg/kg/dose Q 6-12h. *Adult*: 250-750 mg Q 6-12h, max 3 g/d.

	Inj: 50 mg/ml	**IV:** *Child:* 2.5-16.25 mg/kg/dose Q 6-12h. *Adult:* 250-1000 mg Q6h.
Methylene blue	*Inj:* 10 mg/ml	*Child/adult:* 1-2 mg/kg IV over 5min, repeat in 1h prn.
Methylprednisolone (*Medrol, Solu-Medrol*)	*Tab:* 2, 4, 8, 16, 24, 32 mg *Inj:* 40-2000 mg/vial	*Dosage dependent on disease process undergoing treatment.*
Methysergide (*Sansert*)	*Tab:* 2 mg	*Migraine or vascular headache:* *Adult:* 4-8 mg/d po divided TID with meals. Max duration of use is for 6 months.
Metoclopramide (*Reglan*)	*Liquid:* 5, 10 mg/5 ml *Tab:* 5, 10 mg *Inj:* 5 mg/ml	*GE reflux, gastric stasis:* *Child:* 0.05-0.1 mg/kg/dose po/IV Q 6h. *Adult:* 5-20 mg po Q 6h or 10-20 mg IV Q 4-6h prn.
Metocurine iodide (*Metubine*)	*Inj:* 2 mg/ml	*Adult:* 0.2-0.4 mg/kg/dose IV over 30-60sec.
Metolazone (*Zaroxolyn, Diulo*)	*Tab:* 0.5, 2.5, 5, 10 mg	*Adult:* 2.5-20 mg po QD.
Metoprolol (*Lopressor, Toprol XL*)	*Tab:* 50, 100 mg *Tab (XL):* 50, 100, 200 mg *Inj:* 1 mg/ml	*HTN:* *Adult:* 100-450 mg/d po QD or divided BID. XL: 50-400 mg po QD. *Angina:* *Adult:* 100-400 mg/d po divided BID. XL: 100-400 mg po QD. *MI:* see p. 21.
Metronidazole (*Flagyl, Protostat*)	*Tab:* 250, 500 mg *Inj:* 500 mg	**PO:** *Giardia:* p. 13. *Trichomonas:* p. 33. *Bact. vaginosis:* p. 33. **IV:** *Child >1 mo.-adult:* initial dose 15 mg/kg, then 7.5 mg/kg/dose Q 6h, max 4 g/d.

See index for generic names of proprietary meds

Pediatric and Adult Drug Dosing

MEDICATION	PREPARATIONS	DOSING
Mexiletine *(Mexitil)*	Cap: 150, 200, 250 mg	*Adult:* 200-400 mg po Q8h.
Mezlocillin *(Mezlin)*	Inj: 1, 2, 3, 4 g	*Child <7 days:* 75 mg/kg/dose IM/IV Q12h. *Child >7 days:* 75 mg/kg/dose IM/IV. *If ≤2 kg, give Q 8h; if >2 kg, give Q 6h.* *Adult:* 50-75 mg/kg/dose IV Q6h.
Miconazole *(Monistat)*	Vag supp: 100, 200 mg Cream/lotion: 2%	**Vaginal candida:** vag supp in vagina Qhs for 3d (200 mg) or 7d (100 mg). **Tinea corporis, cruris, or pedis and cutaneous candidiasis:** apply cream or lotion BID for 2-3 weeks.
Midazolam *(Versed)*	Inj: 1, 5 mg/ml	**Sedation for procedures:** *Child/adult:* 0.035-0.04 mg/kg IV over 2min. Repeat prn. *For elderly patients, start with 1 mg.* **Sedation for rapid sequence intubation:** *Child/adult:* 0.05-0.15 mg/kg. For RSI protocol see p. 150-151.
Milrinone *(Primacor)*	Inj: 1 mg/ml	**CHF loading dose:** *Adult:* 50 µg/kg IV over 10min. **CHF maintenance infusion:** 0.375-0.75 µg/kg/min IV. Total dose/d = 0.59-1.13 mg/kg.
Minocycline *(Minocin)*	Liquid: 50 mg/5 ml Cap: 50, 100 mg Inj: 100 mg	**PO/IV:** *Child >8 y.o.:* initial dose 4 mg/kg, then 2 mg/kg/dose Q12h. *Adult:* first dose 200 mg, then 100 mg Q12h.

Minoxidil (*Loniten*)	*Tab:* 2.5, 10 mg	*Child <12 y.o.:* start 0.2 mg/kg/dose (max 5 mg) QD. Usual dose 0.25-1.0 mg/kg QD or divided BID. Max 50 mg/d. *Child >12 y.o.-adult:* usual effective dose 5-40 mg po QD. Max 100 mg/d.
Misoprostol (*Cytotec*)	*Tab:* 100, 200 µg	*Adult:* 100-200 µg po QID.
Moricizine (*Ethmozine*)	*Tab:* 200, 250, 300 mg	***Ventricular arrhythmia:** Adult:* 200-300 mg po Q 8h.
Morphine sulfate (*Roxanol, MS-Contin, Oramorph SR, OMS, MSIR, RMS*)	*Tab: Morphine sulfate:* 10, 15, 30 mg; MSIR: 15 mg *Tab (SR):* MS-Contin: 15, 30, 60, 100 mg; Oramorph SR: 30, 60, 100 mg *Liquid: Morphine sulfate* Oral Sltn, Morphine sulfate MSIR: 10, 20 mg/5 ml; Rescudose: 4 mg/ml; Roxanol Conc. Oral Sltn, MSIR Oral Sltn Concentrate, OMS Concentrate, Roxanol 100 Concentrated Oral Solution: 20 mg/ml *Supp:* Morphine sulfate suppositories, RMS, or Roxanol: 5, 10, 20, 30 mg *Inj:* 0.5, 1, 2, 4, 5, 8, 10, 15, 25 mg/ml	**PO:** *Adult (tab, liquid):* 10-30 mg Q 4h. *Adult (tab SR):* 30-100 mg or more as needed BID. **PR:** *Adult:* 10-20 mg Q 4h prn. **SC/IM/IV:** *Child:* 0.1-0.2 mg/kg/dose (max 15 mg) Q 2-4h prn. *Adult:* 5-20 mg Q 4h prn.
Mupirocin (*Bactroban*)	*Ointment:* 2%	*Child/adult:* apply to affected area of skin TID.
Nabumetone (*Relafen*)	*Tab:* 500, 750 mg	*Adult:* start 1000 mg po single dose. Increase to 1500-2000 mg/d po as single dose or divided BID.

Pediatric and Adult Drug Dosing

See index for generic names of proprietary meds

MEDICATION	PREPARATIONS	DOSING
Nadolol (Corgard)	Tab: 20, 40, 80, 120, 160 mg	**HTN:** Adult: 40-320 mg po QD. **Angina:** Adult: 40-240 mg po QD.
Nafcillin (Unipen, Nafil)	Liquid: 250 mg/5 ml Tab: 500 mg Cap: 250 mg Inj: 0.5, 1.0, 2.0 g	**PO:** Child: 50-100 mg/kg/d divided Q 4-6h. Adult: 250-1000 mg Q 4-6h. **IM/IV:** Child <7 days: 50 mg/kg/dose IV Q 12h. Child >7 days: 37.5 mg/kg/dose IV Q 6h. Adult: 1-2 g IM/IV Q 4h.
Nalbuphine (Nubain)	Inj: 10, 20 mg/ml	**SC/IM/IV:** Adult: 10-20 mg Q 3-6h prn.
Nalidixic acid (Negram)	Liquid: 250 mg/5 ml Tab: 250, 500, 1000 mg	Adult: 1 g po Q 6h.
Naloxone (Narcan)	Inj: 0.02, 0.4, 1 mg/ml	**SC/IM/IV:** Child: 0.1 mg/kg/dose. Adult: 0.8-2.0 mg/dose.
Naproxen (Naprosyn)	Liquid: 125 mg/5 ml Tab: 250, 375, 500 mg	Adult: 250-500 mg po BID.
Nedocromil (Tilade)	Inhaler: 1.75 mg/puff	**Asthma prevention:** Children >12 y.o.-adult: 2 puffs Q 6h.

Neomycin	*Liquid:* 125 mg/5 ml *Tab:* 500 mg	***E. coli diarrhea:*** *Child:* 12.5-25 mg/kg/dose Q 6h. *Adult:* 12.5 mg/kg/dose Q 6h for 2-3d. **Hepatic encephalopathy:** 1-3 g po QID.
Neomycin/ polymixin B/ hydrocortisone otic *(Cortisporin)*	*Susp:* Neo 3.5 mg, Poly 10,000 U, Hydro 10 mg/ml	*Child/adult:* 3 drops *(child)* or 4 drops *(adult)* in ear TID-QID.
Neostigmine *(Prostigmin)*	*Inj:* 0.25, 0.5, 1 mg/ml	***Reversal of non-depolarizing paralyzing agents:*** *Child <1 y.o.:* 0.025-0.1 mg/kg/dose IV. *Child >1 y.o.:* 0.025-0.08 mg/kg/dose IV. *Adult:* 1-2 mg IV, may repeat up to 5 mg total IV. *Also give atropine or glycopyrrolate.* ***For emergency treatment of myasthenia:*** see p. 20.
Netilmicin *(Netromycin)*	*Inj:* 10, 25, 100 mg/ml	**IM/IV:** *Child <6 wk:* 5 mg/kg/d divided Q 12h. *Child >6 wk:* 7.5 mg/kg/d divided Q 8h. *Adult:* 4.0-6.5 mg/kg/d divided Q 8-12h. *Alternate QD dosing (adult only):* 6.5 mg/kg.
Nicardipine *(Cardene)*	*Cap:* 20, 30 mg *Cap (SR):* 30, 45, 60 mg *Inj:* 25 mg/10 ml	**PO:** *Adult:* 40-120 mg/d. Divide TID (cap) or BID (SR). **IV:** *Adult:* start infusion at 5 mg/h, increase rate by 2.5 mg/h every 5-15min up to max 15 mg/h. Decrease to 3 mg/h when desired BP obtained.
Niclosamide *(Niclocide)*	*Tab (chew):* 500 mg	***Worms:*** see p. 35.

Pediatric and Adult Drug Dosing

See index for generic names of proprietary meds

MEDICATION	PREPARATIONS	DOSING
Nicotine transdermal (*Habitrol, Nicoderm, Nicotrol, Prostep*)	*Patch:* Habitrol/Nicoderm: 21, 14, 11 mg/d Nicotrol: 15, 10, 5 mg/d Prostep: 22, 11 mg/d	Apply patch to non-hairy part of trunk or upper, outer arm. Habitrol/Nicoderm: one 21 mg patch QD for 6wks, then one 14 mg patch for 2-4wks, then one 7 mg patch for 2-4wks. Nicotrol: one 15 mg patch QD for 4-12wks, then one 10 mg patch for 2-4wks, then one 5 mg patch for 2-4wks. Prostep: one 22 mg patch QD for 4-8wks, then one 11 mg patch for 2-4wks
Nifedipine (*Procardia, Procardia XL, Adalat*)	*Cap:* 10, 20 mg *Cap (XL):* 30, 60, 90 mg	*Adult:* 30-180 mg/d po. Divide TID (tab) or QD (XL). Max XL dose 120 mg/d.
Nimodipine (*Nimotop*)	*Cap:* 30 mg	**Subarachnoid hemorrhage:** *Adult:* 60 mg po Q 4h for 21d.
Nitrofurantoin (*Macrodantin, Macrobid*)	*Liquid:* 25 mg/5 ml *Cap:* 25, 50, 100 mg *Cap (SR)* Macrobid: 100 mg	**UTI treatment:** *Child >1 mo.:* 1.25-1.75 mg/kg/dose po QID. *Adult:* 50-100 mg po QID or (Cap SR) 100 mg po BID. **UTI prophylaxis:** *Child >1 mo.:* 1-2 mg/kg/dose po Q hs. *Adult:* 50-100 mg po Q hs.
Nitroglycerin Subling tab-*Nitrostat*; Tab/Cap-*Nitro-Time, Nitroglyn, Nitrong*; Buccal (transmuco-	*Subling tab:* 0.3, 0.4, 0.6 mg *Tab:* 2.6, 6.5, 9 mg *Cap:* 2.5, 6.5, 9 mg *Buccal tab:* 1, 2, 3 mg	**Subling tab:** 0.15-0.6 mg po prn chest pain or expectation of chest pain Q 5min for 15-30min. **Tab/cap:** 7.5-27 mg/d po divided Q 8-12h. **Buccal tab:** 1 tab Q 3-5h. Place tab between lip and gum above incisors or between cheek and gum.

sa) tab-*Nitrogard*; Spray-*Nitrogard*; Transderm-Minitran, Deponit, Transderm-Nitro, Nitrodisc, Nitrodur, NTS; Ointment-*Nitro-Bid, Nitrol*)	*Transdermal patch*: 0.1, 0.2, 0.3, 0.4, 0.6 mg/h *Lingual spray*: 0.4 mg/spray *Topical ointment*: 2% *Inj*: 0.5, 0.8, 5 mg/ml	**Lingual spray**: 1-2 sprays prn chest pain or expectation of chest pain Q5min for 15-30min. **Transdermal**: 0.1-0.6 mg/h patch on for 12-14h/d and off for 10-12h/d. Generally off while sleeping. **Ointment**: 0.5-5.0 inches to skin Q8h. **IV**: start 5 µg/min infusion with stepwise increases of 10 µg/min Q5min as needed.
Nitroprusside (*Nipride*)	*Inj*: 50 mg vial	*Child/adult*: start at 0.5 µg/kg/min IV, titrate to max 10 µg/kg/min infusion. *See dosing table p. 155.*
Nizatidine (*Axid*)	*Cap*: 150, 300 mg	*Active PUD*: *Adult*: 150 mg po BID or 300 mg po Q.hs. *Maintenance PUD*: 150 mg po Q.hs.
Norfloxacin (*Noroxin*)	*Tab*: 400 mg	*UTI*: *Adult*: 400 mg po BID 1h before or 2h after meals or antacids.
Nortriptyline (*Pamelor*)	*Liquid*: 10 mg/5 ml *Cap*: 10, 25, 50, 75 mg	*Adult*: 75-100 mg po QD or in divided doses.
Nystatin (*Mycostatin*)	*Vag tab*: 100,000 U *Cream/ointment*: 100,000 U/g *Oral susp*: 100,000 U/ml *Tab*: 500,000 U	*Vaginal candida*: vag tab in vagina Qhs for 14d. *Cutaneous/mucocutaneous candida*: apply cream or ointment BID until lesions are healed. *Thrush/candida esophagitis*: *Child <1 y.o.*: 2 ml po QID. *Child >1 y.o.-adult*: 4-6 ml of susp. po QID. Hold in mouth several min before swallowing. HIV pts may use vag tab (or clotrimazole troche) to prolong contact with mucosa. *Intestinal candidiasis*: 500,000 -1,000,000 U po TID.

Pediatric and Adult Drug Dosing

See index for generic names of proprietary meds

MEDICATION	PREPARATIONS	DOSING
Ofloxacin *(Floxin)*	*Tab:* 200, 300, 400 mg *Inj:* 200, 400 mg/vial	**PO:** *Adult >18 y.o.: **Gonorrhea:*** 400 mg single dose. ***Chlamydia:*** 300 mg Q12h for 7d. ***UTI:*** 200 mg Q12h for 3d, 7d, or 10d, based on severity. ***Prostatitis:*** 300 mg Q12h for 6 weeks. ***Respiratory:*** 400 mg Q12h for 10d. ***Skin:*** 400 mg Q12h for 10d. **IV:** *Adult >18 y.o.: **Respiratory:*** 400 mg Q12h. ***UTI:*** 200 mg Q12h. ***Skin:*** 400 mg Q12h.
Omeprazole *(Prilosec)*	*Cap:* 20 mg	*Adult:* 20 mg po QD.
Ondansetron *(Zofran)*	*Tab:* 4, 8 mg *Inj:* 2 mg/ml	**PO:** *Child 4-12 y.o.:* 4 mg Q4h **x** 3 doses, then 4 mg Q 8h. *Child >12 y.o.-adult:* 8 mg Q4h **x** 3 doses, then 8 mg Q 8h. **IV:** *Child >3 y.o.-adult:* 0.15 mg/kg/dose. Give first dose 30min before chemotherapy; further doses 4h and 8h later. Optional dosing: *adult (only):* 32 mg IV 30min PT chemoRx.
Opium tincture **(Laudanum)** **Opium tincture,** **camphorated** **(Paregoric)**	Laudanum: equivalent to morphine 10 mg/ml Paregoric: equivalent to morphine 2 mg, with anise oil 0.2 mg, benzoic acid 20 mg, camphor 20 mg, glycerin 0.2 ml in ethanol to make 5 ml	*Child:* Paregoric: 0.25-0.5 ml/kg/dose po QD-QID. *Adult:* Laudanum 0.3-1 ml po QID (max 6 ml/d); or Paregoric 5-10 ml po BID-QID until diarrhea subsides. *Laudanum contains 25 times more morphine than paregoric.*

Orphenadrine (*Norflex*)	*Tab:* 100 mg *Inj:* 30 mg/ml	*Adult:* 100 mg po BID or 60 mg IM/IV Q 12h.
Orphenadrine/ aspirin/caffeine (*Norgesic, Norgesic Forte*)	*Tab:* Norgesic: Orph 25 mg, ASA 385 mg, Caff 30 mg *Tab:* Norgesic Forte: Orph 50 mg, ASA 770 mg, Caff 60 mg	*Adult:* Norgesic 1-2 tabs po Q 6-8h. Norgesic Forte: 1 tab po Q 6-8h.
Oxacillin (*Bactocil, Prostaphlin*)	*Liquid:* 250 mg/5 ml *Cap:* 250, 500 mg *Inj:* 0.25, 0.5, 1, 2, 4 g	**PO:** *Child:* 12-25 mg/kg/dose Q 6h. *Adult:* 0.5-1.0 g Q 6h. **IM/IV:** *Child:* 37.5 mg/kg/dose Q 6h. *Adult:* 1-2 g Q 4-6h.
Oxaprozin (*Daypro*)	*Tab:* 600 mg	*Adult:* 600-1200 mg po QD.
Oxybutynin (*Ditropan*)	*Liquid:* 5 mg/5 ml *Tab:* 5 mg	*Child >5 y.o.:* 5 mg po BID-TID. *Adult:* 5 mg po BID-QID.
Oxycodone (*Roxicodone*)	*Liquid:* 5 mg/5 ml, 20 mg/ml *Tab:* 5 mg *Supp:* 10, 20 mg	**PO:** *Child:* 0.05-0.15 mg/kg/dose Q 4-6h, max 10 mg/dose. *Adult:* 5 mg Q 3-6h. **PR:** *Adult:* 10-40 mg TID-QID.
Oxycodone/ acetaminophen (*Tylox, Percocet, Roxilox*)	*Liquid:* Oxy 5 mg, Acet 325 mg/5 ml *Cap:* Oxy 5 mg, Acet 500 mg *Tab:* Oxy 5 mg, Acet 325 mg; Oxy 5 mg, Acet 500 mg	*Adult:* 1 tab, 1 cap, or 5 ml po Q 6h prn.

Pediatric and Adult Drug Dosing

See index for generic names of proprietary meds

MEDICATION	PREPARATIONS	DOSING
Oxycodone/aspirin (*Percodan, Roxiprin, Codoxy*)	*Tab:* Oxy 2.44 mg, ASA 325 mg; Oxy 4.88 mg, ASA 325 mg	*Child 6-12 y.o.:* ¼ tab po Q6h prn. *Child >12 y.o.:* ½ tab po Q6h prn. *Adult:* 1-2 caps po Q6h prn.
Pancuronium (*Pavulon*)	*Inj:* 1, 2 mg/ml	***Defasciculating/priming:*** *Child/adult:* 0.01 mg/kg/dose IV. ***Paralyzing dose:*** *Child <1 mo.:* 0.02 mg/kg/dose IV. *Child >1 mo.-adult:* 0.04-0.1 mg/kg/dose IV.
Paregoric		See p. 84.
Paroxetine (*Paxil*)	*Tab:* 20, 30 mg	*Adult:* 20-50 mg po QD.
Penicillin G	*Inj:* 200,000, 500,000, 1 million, 5 million, 10 million, 20 million U	*Child <7 days:* **Meningitis:** 100,000-150,000 U/kg/d IM/IV divided Q 8-12h. *Child 7 days-1 y.o.:* **Meningitis:** 150,000-250,000 U/kg/d IM/IV divided Q6-8h. *Child >1 y.o.:* **Meningitis:** 250,000 U/kg/d IM/IV divided Q3-4h. *Child <7 days:* **Other:** 50,000 U/kg/d IM/IV divided Q 12h. *Child >7 days:* **Other:** 75,000 U/kg/d IM/IV divided Q8h. *Adult, low dose (LD):* 4-6 MU/d IV divided Q 4-6h *Adult, medium dose (MD):* 8-12 MU/d IV divided Q 4-6h. *Adult, high dose (HD):* 12-30 MU/d IV divided Q 3-4h.

Penicillin V	*Liquid:* 125 mg (200,000 U), 250 mg (400,000 U)/5 ml *Tab:* 125, 250, 500 mg	*Child:* 6-12 mg/kg/dose po Q 6h. *Adult:* 250-500 mg po Q 6h.
Pentamidine *(NebuPent,* *Pentam 300)*	*Sltn for inhalation:* 300 mg *Inj:* 300 mg	***Pneumocystis treatment and prophylaxis:*** see p. 24-25.
Pentazocine *(Talwin)*	*Tab:* 50 mg with naloxone 0.5 mg *Inj:* 30 mg/ml	**PO:** *Adult:* 50-100 mg Q 3-4h, max 600 mg/d. **SC/IM:** *Adult:* 30-60 mg Q 3-4h, max 360 mg/d. **IV:** *Adult:* 30 mg Q 3h prn.
Pentobarbital *(Nembutal)*	*Inj:* 50 mg/ml	**Sedation:** *Child:* 1-3 mg/kg IV, max 100 mg/d. *Adult:* 100-200 mg IV at 50 mg/min. Additional doses Q 1-5min to max 500 mg.
Pentoxifylline *(Trental)*	*Tab:* 400 mg	*Adult:* 400 mg po Q 8-12h.
Permethrin *(Elimite, Nix)*	*Cream:* tube 60 g of 5% *Creme rinse:* 2 fluid oz of 1%	**Lice:** see p. 16. **Scabies:** see p. 28.
Perphenazine *(Trilafon)*	*Tab:* 2, 4, 8, 16 mg *Liquid:* 16 mg/5 ml *Inj:* 5 mg/ml	**Psychosis:** **PO:** *Adult:* 4-16 mg BID-QID. **IM:** *Adult:* 5 mg Q 6h prn.
Phenazopyridine *(Pyridium, Di-Azo)*	*Tab:* 100, 200 mg	*Child:* 4 mg/kg/dose po TID. *Adult:* 100-200 mg po TID.

Pediatric and Adult Drug Dosing

See index for generic names of proprietary meds

MEDICATION	PREPARATIONS	DOSING
Phenelzine (*Nardil*)	*Tab:* 15 mg	***Initiation:*** *Adult:* 45-90 mg/d divided TID-QID for 2-6wk. ***Maintenance:*** *Adult:* 15 mg QD or QOD.
Phenobarbital (*Barbita, Solfoton, Luminal*)	*Liquid:* 15, 20 mg/5 ml *Tab:* 8, 15, 16, 30, 32 60, 65, 100 mg *Cap:* 16 mg *Inj:* 30, 60, 65, 130 mg/ml	***IV loading dose:*** *Child/adult:* 15-20 mg/kg at 50 mg/min. ***PO maintenance:*** *Child <1 month:* 3-5 mg/kg QD or div BID. *Child 1 mo.-1 y.o.:* 5-6 mg/kg QD or div BID. *Child 1-5 y.o.:* 6-8 mg/kg QD or div BID. *Child 6-12 y.o.:* 4-6 mg/kg QD or div BID. *Child >12 y.o. -adult:* 1-3 mg/kg QD or div BID.
Phenobarbital/ ergotamine/ belladonna (*Bellergal-S*)	*Tab:* Phenobarbital 40 mg, Ergotamine 0.6 mg, Belladonna 0.2 mg	*Adult:* 1 tab po BID.
Phenobarbital/ hyoscyamine/ atropine/scopola- mine (*Donnatal*)	*Tab/Cap/Liquid per 5 ml:* Phen 16.2 mg, Hyos 0.1037 mg, Atro 0.0194 mg, Scop 0.0065 mg	*Child:* 0.10 ml/kg/dose po Q 4h. *Adult:* 1-2 tab(s) or cap(s) or 5-10 ml po TID-QID.
Phenylbutazone (*Butazolidin*)	*Tab/Cap:* 100 mg	*Adult:* 100-200 mg po TID.
Phenytoin (*Dilantin*)	*Tab (chew):* 50 mg *Cap:* 30, 100 mg	***IV loading:*** *Child/adult:* 15-18 mg/kg at 25-30 mg/min, in emergencies max infusion rate 50 mg/min.

	Cap (ext rel): 30, 100 mg Susp: 30, 125 mg/5 ml Inj: 50 mg/ml	**Seizure maintenance:** *Child:* 4-8 mg/kg/d divided Q 8-12h. *Adult:* 300-600 (usually 300) mg/d divided Q 8-24h. Give extended release form QD only.
Pindolol (*Visken*)	Tab: 5, 10 mg	*Adult:* 10-60 mg/d po divided Q 8-12h.
Piperacillin (*Pipracil*)	Inj: 2, 3, 4 g	*Child >2 mo:* 75 mg/kg/dose IV Q 6h. *Adult:* 2-3 g IV 4-6h.
Piperacillin/ tazobactam (*Zosyn*)	Inj: Pip 2 g, Tazo 0.25 g; Pip 3 g, Tazo 0.375 g; Pip 4 g, Tazo 0.5 g	*Child >12 y.o.-adult:* as piperacillin 3 g IV Q 6h or 4 g IV Q 8h over 30min.
Pirbuterol (*Maxair*)	Inhaler: 200 µg/puff	*Child >12 y.o.-adult:* 1-2 puffs Q 4-6h.
Piroxicam (*Feldene*)	Tab: 10, 20 mg	*Adult:* 20-40 mg/d po QD or divided BID. Elderly start at 10 mg po QD.
Polyethylene glycol (*GoLYTELY*)	*Powder* for oral solution	**Drug OD:** *Child:* 25-40 ml/kg/h po until rectal effluent clear. *Adult:* 240 ml every 10min po until rectal effluent clear or 4 liters have been consumed.
Pralidoxime (*Protopam*)	Inj: 1 g/vial; 600 mg/auto-injector	**Carbamate OD:** see p. 129. **Organophosphate OD:** see p. 131
Pravastatin (*Pravachol*)	Tab: 10, 20, 40 mg	*Adult:* start 10-20 mg po Q hs. Adjust dosage Q 4wk based on response. Max 40 mg/d.
Praziquantel (*Biltricide, Cesol*)	Tab: 600 mg	**Worms:** see p. 35.

Pediatric and Adult Drug Dosing

See index for generic names of proprietary meds

MEDICATION	PREPARATIONS	DOSING
Prazosin (*Minipress*)	*Cap:* 1, 2, 5 mg	*Adult:* initial dose 1 mg BID to TID po, usual maintenance 6-15 mg/d, max 20 mg/d.
Prednisone	*Oral sltn:* 5 mg/ml; 5 mg/ 5 ml *Syrup:* 5 mg/5ml *Tab:* 1, 2.5, 5, 10, 20, 25, 50 mg	*Dosage dependent on disease process undergoing treatment.*
Primidone (*Mysoline*)	*Liquid:* 250 mg/5 ml *Tab:* 50, 250 mg	*Seizure maintenance: Child <8 y.o.:* 10-25 mg/kg/d divided Q6-8h. *Child >8 y.o.-adult:* 0.75-2 g/d divided Q6-8h.
Probenecid (*Benemid*)	*Tab:* 500 mg	*Gout maintenance: Adult:* start 250 mg po BID for 1 week, then 500 mg BID, then adjust dose to max 3 g/d.
Probucol (*Lorelco*)	*Tab:* 250, 500 mg	*Adult:* 500 mg po BID with morning and evening meals.
Procainamide (*Pronestyl, Procan*)	*Cap:* 250, 375, 500 mg *Tab SR:* 250, 500, 750, 1000 mg *Inj:* 100, 500 mg/ml	**PO:** *Child:* 15-50 mg/kg/d divided Q3-6h. Max 4 g/d. *Adult:* 50 mg/kg/d div Q3h (cap/tab) or Q6h (tab SR). **IV:** *Child:* 2-6 mg/kg over 5min, then maintenance drip at 0.020-0.080 mg/kg/min. Max 2 g/d. *Adult:* 20 mg/min up to 1 g, or until arrhythmia resolves, hypotension, or QRS 150% of initial width.

Prochlorperazine (*Compazine*)	*Liquid:* 5 mg/5 ml *Tab:* 5, 10, 25 mg *Tab SR:* 10, 15, 30 mg *Cap (SR):* 10, 15, 30 mg *Supp:* 2.5, 5, 25 mg *Inj:* 5 mg/ml	**PO:** *Child >9 kg and >2 y.o.:* 0.1 mg/kg/dose Q 6h. *Adult:* 5-10 mg Q 6-8h (SR 10-30 mg QD). **PR:** *Child >9 kg and >2 y.o.:* 0.1 mg/kg/dose Q 6h. *Adult:* 25 mg Q 12h. **IM/IV:** *Child >9 kg and >2 y.o.:* 0.13 mg/kg/dose Q 6h. *Adult:* 2.5-10 mg Q 6h.
Promethazine (*Phenergan*)	*Liquid:* 6.25, 25 mg/5 ml *Tab:* 12.5, 25, 50 mg *Supp:* 12.5, 25, 50 mg *Inj:* 25, 50 mg/ml	**PO/PR/IM/IV:** *Child:* 0.25-0.5 mg/kg/dose Q 4-6h. *Adult:* 12.5-25 mg Q 4-6h.
Propafenone (*Rythmol*)	*Tab:* 150, 225, 300 mg	***Ventricular arrhythmias:*** *Adult:* 150-300 mg po Q 8h.
Propoxyphene (*Darvon*)	*Tab:* 65 mg	*Adult:* 1 tab po Q 4h prn.
Propoxyphene/aceta-minophen (*Darvocet, Wygesic*)	*Tab:* Darvocet-N 50: Prop 50, Acet 325 mg; Darvocet-N 100: Prop 100, Acet 650 mg; Wygesic: Prop 65, Acet 650 mg	*Adult:* 1 tab po Q 4h prn.
Propranolol (*Inderal*)	*Liquid:* 20, 40 mg/5 ml; 80 mg/ml *Tab:* 10, 20, 40, 60, 80, 90 mg *Cap (SR):* 60, 80, 120, 160 mg *Inj:* 1 mg/ml	**PO:** *Child:* 1-4 mg/kg/d divided BID-QID. *Adult:* **HTN:** 160-640 mg/d divided BID, TID, or QID (SR QD only). **Angina:** 30-240 mg/d TID-QID (SR QD only). **IV:** *Child:* 0.01-0.1 mg/kg/dose (max 1 mg) Q 6h prn. *Adult:* 1.0 mg Q 5min to desired effect (max total 5 mg).

Pediatric and Adult Drug Dosing

See index for generic names of proprietary meds

MEDICATION	PREPARATIONS	DOSING
Prostaglandin E₁	*Inj*: 500 µg/ml	*Child <1 mo.*: start 0.05-0.1 µg/kg/min IV, advance to 0.2 µg/kg/min IV as needed. When PaO2 increases, decrease to lowest effective dose.Monitor respirations.
Protamine sulfate	*Inj*: 10 mg/ml	*Child/adult*: 1 mg for each 100 U heparin to be reversed over 1-3min IV, max 50 mg over any 10min. Same dose for heparin from either lung tissue or intestinal mucosa.
Pseudoephedrine (*Sudafed*)	*Tab*: 30, 60 mg *Liquid*: 30 mg/5 ml	*Child*: 1 mg/kg/dose po Q 6h. *Adult*: 30-60 mg po Q 4-6h.
Pyrantel pamoate (*Antiminth*)	*Liquid*: 50 mg/ml	**Worms:** see p. 35.
Pyrazinamide	*Tab*: 500 mg	**TB**: *Child*: 15-30 mg/kg/d po QD or divided BID, max 2 g/d. *Adult*: 20-35 mg/kg/dose po QD, max 3 g/d.
Pyrethrins with piperonyl butoxide (*RID*)	*Shampoo*: 2, 4, 8 fl oz	*Lice*: see p. 16.
Pyrimethamine (*Daraprim*)	*Tab*: 25 mg	**Toxoplasmosis:** see p. 31. Pyrimethamine with sulfadoxine: see p. 96.
Quinacrine (*Atabrine*)	*Tab*: 100 mg	**Giardia:** see p. 13.

Quinapril (*Accupril*)	*Tab:* 5, 10, 20, 40 mg	*Adult:* 5-80 mg/d QD or divided BID.
Quinidine gluconate (*Quinaglute*)	*Tab:* 324 mg *Inj:* 80 mg/ml	**PO:** *Adult:* 324-660 mg Q 8-12h. **IM:** *Adult:* start 600 mg, then 400 mg Q 2h to desired result. **IV:** *Adult:* 800 mg in 40 cc D5W at 16 mg/min; stop if QRS widens, HR <120 BPM, or sinus rhythm resumes.
Quinidine polygalacturonate (*Cardioquin*)	*Tab:* 275 mg	*To terminate arrhythmias: Adult:* start 1-3 tabs Q 3-4h x 3-4 doses. If no effect, increase dose by ½-1 tab and repeat Q 3-4h for 3-4 doses. *Maintenance: Adult:* 1 tab BID-TID.
Quinidine sulfate (*Quinidex*)	*Tab:* 200, 300 mg *Tab* (Quinidex Extentab): 300 mg	**PO:** *Maintenance: Child:* 3.75-15 mg/kg/dose Q 6h. *Adult: To terminate arrhythmias:* 200-600 mg Q 1-4h until desired effect. *Maintenance:* 300-600 mg Q 6h. (Quinidex Extentabs: 300-600 Q 8-12h.)
Quinine	*Tab:* 260, 325 mg *Cap:* 130, 200, 300, 325 mg	*Malaria: Child:* 6.3 mg/kg/dose po Q 8h, max 650 mg/dose. *Adult:* 650 mg po Q 8h.
Rabies immune globulin	*Inj:* 150 IU/ml	**Rabies prophylaxis:** see p. 27 and p.140, and rabies vaccine below.
Rabies vaccine	*Inj:* Human diploid cell (HDCV) and rabies adsorbed (RVA): 2.5 IU/IM vial	**Rabies prophylaxis:** see p. 27 and p.140, and rabies immune globulin above.

Pediatric and Adult Drug Dosing

See index for generic names of proprietary meds

MEDICATION	PREPARATIONS	DOSING
Ramipril *(Altace)*	*Tab:* 1.25, 2.5, 5, 10 mg	*Adult:* 2.5-20 mg/d po QD or divided BID.
Ranitidine *(Zantac)*	*Liquid:* 15 mg/ml *Tab:* 150, 300 mg *Inj:* 25 mg/ml	**PO:** *Child:* 1-2 mg/kg/dose BID. *Adult:* 150 mg BID or 150-300 mg at hs. **IV:** *Child:* 1-2 mg/kg/d divided Q 6-8h. *Adult:* 50 mg Q 6-8h.
Ribavirin *(Virazole)*	*Inhalation sltn:* 6 g/100 ml	**Aerosol:** *Child:* dilute 6 g in 300 ml sterile water for 20 mg/ml solution. Administer over 12-18h QD for 3-7d.
Rifabutin *(Ansamycin,* *Mycobutin)*	*Cap:* 150 mg	**Prevention of disseminated *Mycobacterium avium* complex in advanced AIDS:** 300 mg QD. If patient likely to have GI upset, use 150 mg BID.
Rifampin *(Rifadin)*	*Cap:* 150, 300 mg *Inj:* 600 mg/vial	**TB:** *Child* >5 y.o.: 10-20 mg/kg/dose (max 600 mg) po/IV QD or same dose po twice/week 1h before or 2h after any meal. *Adult:* 600 mg po/IV QD or same dose twice/wk po 1h before or 2h after any meal. ***Staph. aureus/epidermidis:*** *Adult:* 150-300 mg po QID with other agents. ***Meningitis prophylaxis:*** see p. 19.
Rimantadine *(Flumadine)*	*Tab:* 100 mg *Liquid:* 50 mg/ml	*Child <20 kg:* 5 mg/kg po QD or divided BID. *Child >20 kg–adult:* 100 mg po QD or divided BID.

Salsalate *(Disalcid)*	*Cap:* 500 mg *Tab:* 500, 750 mg	*Adult:* 3 g/d divided BID, TID, or QID, and taken prn.
Scopolamine *(Transderm Scop)*	*Transderm patch:* 1.5 mg	*Adult:* apply patch behind the ear 4h prior to time anti-emetic action is required. Duration of action: 72h.
Selenium sulfide *(Selsun)*	*Lotion:* 1, 2.5%	*Child (only):* **Tinea versicolor:** apply weekly for 4 weeks. **Tinea capitis:** apply twice weekly for 2-4 weeks. **Tinea:** see p. 30. Apply to affected area for 10min, rinse.
Sertraline *(Zoloft)*	*Tab:* 50,100 mg	*Adult:* 50-200 mg po QD.
Silver sulfadiazine *(Silvadene)*	*Cream 1%:* 20, 50, 85, 400, 1000 g	*Child >2 mo.-adult:* apply QD-BID to debrided burns.
Simethicone *(Gas-X, Mylicon)*	*Tab (chew):* 40, 80, 125 mg *Tab (SR):* 60, 95 mg	*Child >12 y.o.-adult:* 40-125 mg QID after meals and at hs as needed.
Simvastatin *(Zocor)*	*Tab:* 5, 10, 20, 40 mg	*Adult:* start 5-10 mg po each evening. Adjust Q 4wk depending on pt response and tolerance. Max 40 mg/d.
Sodium polystyrene sulfonate *(Kayexalate)*	*Liquid:* 15 g/60 ml *Powder:* 3.5 g/5 ml	*Child:* 1 g/kg/dose po or as retention enema Q2-6h. *Adult:* 15-60 g po or 30-50 g as retention enema Q2-6h.
Sotalol *(Betapace)*	*Tab:* 80, 160, 240 mg	*Adult:* start 80 mg po BID. Dose may be increased Q 2-3d to max 320 mg/d divided BID or TID.
Spectinomycin *(Trobicin)*	*Inj:* 2, 4 g	**Gonorrhea:** see p. 13-14.

Pediatric and Adult Drug Dosing

See index for generic names of proprietary meds

MEDICATION	PREPARATIONS	DOSING
Spironolactone (*Aldactone*)	*Tab:* 25, 50, 100 mg	*Child:* 1.0-3.3 mg/kg/d po divided Q 6-12h. *Adult:* 25-200 mg/d po divided Q 6-12h.
Streptokinase (*Streptase*)	*Inj:* 250,000 U; 750,000 U; 1,500,000 U	**Venous thrombosis, deep:** see p. 34. **Myocardial infarction:** see p. 20. **Pulmonary embolus:** see p. 27.
Succinylcholine (*Anectine*)	*Inj:* 20, 50, 100 mg/ml	**Paralysis for rapid sequence intubation:** *Child/adult:* 1.0-1.5 mg/kg/dose IV. See p. 150-151 for RSI protocol.
Sucralfate (*Carafate*)	*Tab:* 1 g	*Child >12 y.o.-adult:* 1 g po QID 1h before meals and at hs.
Sulfadiazine (*Microsulfon*)	*Tab:* 500 mg	Dose varies with disease. **Toxoplasmosis:** see p. 31.
Sulfadoxine/ pyrimethamine (*Fansidar*)	*Tab:* Sulfadoxine 500 mg, pyrimethamine 25 mg	**Malaria attack:** *Child <4 y.o.:* ³/₄ tab po. *Child 4-8 y.o.:* 1¹/₂ tab po. *Child 9-15 y.o.:* 2¹/₄ tabs po. *Child >15 y.o.-adult:* 3 tabs po. Single dose only. Give with or without quinine. **Malaria prophylaxis:** *Child <4 y.o.:* ¹/₄ tab po Q wk. *Child 4-8 y.o.:* ¹/₂ tab po Q wk. *Child 9-14 y.o.:* ³/₄ tab po Q wk. *Child >14 y.o.-adult:* 1 tab po Q wk. May double dose and give Q 2wk.

Drug	Forms	Dosage
Sulfamethoxazole (*Gantanol*)	*Liquid:* 500 mg/5 ml *Tab:* 500, 1000 mg	***UTI:*** *Child:* initial dose 50-60 mg/kg po, then 25-30 mg/kg/dose po BID. Max 75 mg/kg/d. *Adult:* initial dose 2 g po, then 1 g po BID.
Sulfasalazine (*Azulfidine*)	*Liquid:* 250 mg/5 ml *Tab:* 500 mg	***Maintenance:*** *Child >2 y.o.:* 30 mg/kg/d po divided Q 6h. *Adult:* 1.5-2.0 g/d po divided Q 6h.
Sulfisoxazole (*Gantrisin*)	*Liquid:* 500 mg/5 ml *Tab:* 500 mg	*Child >2 mo.:* initial dose 75 mg/kg po, then 37.5 mg/kg/dose po Q 6h. *Adult:* initial dose 2-4 g po, then 1-2 g po Q 6h.
Sulindac (*Clinoril*)	*Tab:* 150, 200 mg	*Adult:* 150-200 mg po Q 12h.
Sumatriptan (*Imitrex*)	*Inj:* 6 mg in 1 ml syringe; 6 mg in 2 ml unit dose	***Migraine HA:*** 6 mg SC. No evidence second injection will work if first fails. Max 2 doses (12 mg) per 24h must be separated by at least 1h. *Do not use immediately after ergot.*
Tacrine (*Cognex*)	*Cap:* 10, 20, 30, 40 mg	*Adult:* 10-40 mg po QID.
Terazosin (*Hytrin*)	*Tab:* 1, 2, 5 mg	*Adult:* 1-5 mg/d po QD or divided BID.
Terbinafine (*Lamisil*)	*Cream 1%:* 15, 30 g containers	*Child >12 y.o.-adult:* apply to affected and immediately surrounding area BID until improved. Minimum duration 7d, maximum 28d.

Pediatric and Adult Drug Dosing

MEDICATION	PREPARATIONS	DOSING
Terbutaline *(Breathine, Bricanyl)*	*Tab:* 2.5, 5 mg *Inhaler:* 200 µg/puff *Inj:* 1 mg/ml (1:1000)	**PO:** *Child <12 y.o.:* 0.05 mg/kg/dose initially, increase as necessary to max 0.15 mg/kg/dose TID or max 5 mg/d. *Child 12-15 y.o.-adult:* 2.5 mg po TID. *Child >15 y.o.-adult:* 5 mg TID. **Inhaler:** *Child/adult:* 2 puffs Q4-6h. **Nebulization:** *Child <2 y.o.:* 0.5 mg in 2.5 ml NS. *Child 2-9 y.o.:* 1 mg in 2.5 ml NS. *Child >9 y.o.-adult:* 1.5 mg in 2.5 ml NS. **SC:** *Child <12 y.o.:* 0.005-0.01 mg/kg/dose Q 15-20min up to 3 doses, max 0.4 mg/dose. *Child >12 y.o.-adult:* 0.25 mg, may repeat in 15-30min, max 0.5 mg in 4h.
Terconazole *(Terazol 3, Terazol 7)*	*Vag cream:* 0.4, 0.8% in 45 g tubes with applicator *Vag supp:* 80 mg	*Adult:* one applicator-full (cream 0.8%) or suppository intravaginally Q hs for 3d, or one applicator-full (cream 0.4%) Q hs for 7d.
Terfenadine *(Seldane)*	*Tab:* 60 mg	*Child 3-6 y.o.:* 15 mg/dose po BID. *Child 7-12 y.o.:* 30 mg/dose po BID. *Child >12 y.o.-adult:* 60 mg/dose po BID.
Tetanus immune globulin *(Hyper-Tet)*	*Inj:* 250 U/vial	**Prevention:** *Child/adult:* 250-500 U IM. Also see p. 133. **Treatment:** *Child/adult:* 3000-6000 U IM. *Give at different site from toxoid.*

Drug	Formulations	Dosing
Tetracycline	Liquid: 125, 250 mg/5 ml; Tab: 250, 500 mg; Cap: 100, 250, 500 mg	*Child >8 y.o.:* 6-12 mg/kg/dose po Q 6h. *Adult:* 250-500 mg/dose po Q 6h.
Thiabendazole (*Mintezol*)	Liquid: 500 mg/5 ml; Tab (chew): 500 mg	**Worms:** see p. 35.
Thiamine	Inj: 100, 200 mg/ml	*Wernicke's encephalopathy: Adult:* 100 mg IV, then 50-100 mg IM/IV QD.
Thiethylperazine (*Torecan, Norzine*)	Tab: 10 mg; Supp: 10 mg; Inj: 5 mg/ml	**PO/PR/IM:** *Child >12 y.o.-adult:* 10 mg Q 8h prn.
Thiopental (*Pentothal*)	Syringes: 250, 400, 500 mg; Inj: 0.5, 1.0 g/vial	*Rapid sequence intubation: Child/adult:* 2-5 mg/kg/dose IV. Use smaller dose if patient at risk for hemodynamic compromise. See p. 150-151 for rapid sequence intubation protocol.
Thioridazine (*Mellaril*)	Liquid: 25, 100/5 ml; 30, 100 mg/ml; Tab: 10, 15, 25, 50, 100, 150, 200 mg	*Adult:* 200-800 mg/d po divided BID-QID. Usual dose 50-100 mg po TID.
Thiothixene (*Navane*)	Liquid: 5 mg/ml; Cap: 1, 2, 5, 10, 20 mg; Inj: 2, 5 mg/ml	**PO:** *Adult:* start 2 mg TID, usual maintenance 2-20 mg BID-TID. **IM:** *Adult:* 4 mg BID-QID.
Ticarcillin (*Ticar*)	Inj: 1, 3, 6 g	**IV:** *Child <7 days:* 150-225 mg/kg/d divided Q 8-12h. *Child >7 days:* 225-300 mg/kg/d divided Q 4-6h. *Adult:* 3.0 g Q 3-6h (or 250-300 mg/kg/d divided Q 3-6h).

Pediatric and Adult Drug Dosing

See index for generic names of proprietary meds

MEDICATION	PREPARATIONS	DOSING
Ticarcillin clavulanate (*Timentin*)	*Inj:* ticarcillin 3 g, clavulanic acid 100 mg	*IV: Child <7 days:* 150-225 mg/kg/d divided Q 8-12h. *Child >7 days:* 225-300 mg/kg/d divided Q 4-6h. *Adult:* 3.1 g Q 4-6h.
Ticlopidine (*Ticlid*)	*Tab:* 250 mg	*Adult:* 250 mg po BID.
Timolol (*Blocadren*)	*Tab:* 5, 10, 20 mg	*HTN: Adult:* 10-30 mg po BID. *Post MI: Adult:* 10 mg po BID. *Angina: Adult:* 5-15 mg po TID.
Tioconazole (*Vagistat*)	*Vag ointment:* 6.5% in 4.6 g applicator	*Adult:* one applicator-full (300 mg) at hs once only.
Tobramycin (*Nebcin*)	*Inj:* 10, 40 mg/ml	*IM/IV: Child <7 days:* 4 mg/kg/d divided Q 12h. *Child >7 days-1 y.o.:* 6 mg/kg/d divided Q 8h. *Child >1 y.o.:* 4-5 mg/kg/d divided Q 8h. *Adult:* load 2 mg/kg, then 1.7 mg/kg Q 8h. *Alternate QD dosing:* 5.1 mg/kg.
Tocainide (*Tonocard*)	*Tab:* 400, 600 mg	*Adult:* 400-800 mg po Q 8h.
Tolazamide (*Ronase, Tolinase*)	*Tab:* 100, 250, 500 mg	*Adult:* if FBS <200 mg/dl or pt >65 y.o., start 100 mg po QD with breakfast. If FBS >200 mg/dl and pt <65 y.o., start 250 mg po QD. Max 500 mg po BID with meals.

Tolbutamide *(Orinase)*	*Tab:* 250, 500 mg	*Adult:* start 1-2 g po QD or divided BID, adjust to max 3 g/d.
Tolmetin *(Tolectin)*	*Tab:* 200 mg *Tab (coated):* 600 mg *Cap:* 400 mg	*Child >2 y.o.:* start 20 mg/kg, then 15-30 mg/kg/d po divided TID or QID. *Adult:* 400 mg/dose po TID or QID, or 600 mg po TID.
Tranylcypromine *(Parnate)*	*Tab:* 10 mg	*Adult:* 30-60 mg/d po divided BID-TID.
Triamcinolone *(Azmacort)*	*Inhaler:* 100 µg/puff	*Child >6 y.o.:* 1-2 puffs Q 6-8h. *Adult:* 2-4 puffs Q 6-8h.
Triamterene *(Dyrenium)*	*Cap:* 50, 100 mg	*Adult:* 100-150 mg po QD or divided BID.
Triazolam *(Halcion)*	*Tab:* 0.125, 0.25 mg	*Adult <65 y.o.:* 0.125-0.5 mg po at hs for up to 10d. *Adult >65 y.o.:* 0.125-0.25 mg po at hs for up to 10d.
Trifluoperazine *(Stelazine)*	*Tab:* 1, 2, 5, 10 mg *Liquid:* 10 mg/ml *Inj:* 2 mg/ml	**PO:** *Adult:* 7.5-10 mg BID. **IM:** *Adult:* 1-2 mg Q 4-6h prn.
Trimethadione *(Tridione)*	*Liquid:* 200 mg/5 ml *Tab:* 150 mg *Cap:* 300 mg	*Child:* 20-50 mg/kg/d divided TID-QID. Usual maintenance 40 mg/kg/d, max 900 mg/d. *Adult:* 300-600 mg po Q 6-8h.

Pediatric and Adult Drug Dosing

See index for generic names of proprietary meds

MEDICATION	PREPARATIONS	DOSING
Trimethobenzamide *(Tigan)*	Cap: 100, 250 mg Supp: 100, 200 mg Inj: 100 mg/ml	**PO:** *Child 15-40 kg:* 100-200 mg TID-QID. *Child >40 kg-adult:* 250 mg TID-QID. **Rectal:** *Child <15 kg:* 100 mg TID-QID. *Child 15-40 kg:* 100-200 mg TID-QID. *Adult:* 200 mg TID-QID. **IM:** *Adult:* 200 mg TID-QID.
Trimethoprim *(Trimpex)*	*Tab:* 100, 200 mg	*Child >12 y.o.-adult:* 100 mg po BID or 200 mg po QD.
Trimetrexate	*Inj:* 25 mg	*Pneumocystis pneumonia:* see p. 24.
Trimethoprim/ sulfamethoxazole *(Bactrim, Septra)*	*Liquid:* Trimeth 40, Sulf 200 mg/5 ml *Tab:* Trimeth 80 mg, Sulf 400 mg (SS); Trimeth 160, Sulf 800 mg (DS) *Inj:* Trimeth 80, Sulf 400 mg/5 ml	*Pneumocystis pneumonia:* see p. 24. *Pneumocystis pneumonia prophylaxis:* see p. 25. *Minor infections: Child:* 3.75-4.0 mg/kg/dose po Q 12h. *Adult:* as trimeth 160 mg (1 DS) po BID. *Severe infection (UTI): Child/adult:* as trimeth 4-5 mg/kg/dose po/IV Q 12h. *Severe infection (other): Child/adult:* as trimeth 20 mg/kg/d IV divided Q 6-8h.
Valproic acid *(Depakene, Depakote)*	*Cap:* 250 mg *Liquid:* 250 mg/5 ml *Tab SR* (Depakote): 125, 250, 500 mg	*Seizure maintenance: Child/adult:* 15-60 mg/kg/d divided Q 8-12h (give SR form Q 12h only).

Vancomycin *(Vancocin)*	*Inj:* 0.5, 1, 5 g	**PO:** *Pseudomembranous colitis:* see p. 12. *IV: Child <1 month:* initial dose 15 mg/kg, then 10 mg/kg/dose Q 8h. *Child >1 month:* 10 mg/kg/dose Q 6h. *Adult:* 1 g Q 12h.
Vecuronium *(Norcuron)*	*Inj:* 10, 20 mg	*Paralysis for rapid sequence intubation: Child >7 wk-adult:* 0.1-0.15 mg/kg/dose. See p. 150-151 for RSI protocol.
Verapamil *(Calan, Isoptin, Verelan)*	*Tab:* 40, 80, 120 mg SR tab or *cap:* 120, 180, 240 mg *Inj:* 2.5 mg/ml	**PO:** *Child:* 4-10 mg/kg/d divided Q 8h. *Adult:* **HTN:** 240-480 mg/d. Give tab TID, SR tab QD-BID, SR capsule QD only. *Angina/prevention of PSVT:* 240-480 mg/d, divided Q 6-8h, tab only. *Control of ventricular rate in atrial flutter/atrial fibrillation:* 240-320 mg/d, divided Q 6-8h, tab only. *IV: Child <1 y.o.:* 0.1-0.2 mg/kg/dose (0.75-2.0 mg), repeat 10-30min prn. *Child 1-15 y.o.:* 0.1-0.3 mg/kg/dose (2-5 mg), repeat in 10-30min prn. *Adult:* 5-10 mg, repeat 10-30min prn.
Vitamin K1 (Phytonadione) *(Aqua-Mephyton Mephyton, Konakion)*	*Tab:* 5 mg *Inj:* 2, 10 mg/ml	*Vitamin K deficiency: Child:* 1-2 mg IV or 2-5 mg/d po. *Adult:* 5-25 mg po/d. *Oral anticoagulant OD: Child <1 y.o.:* 1 mg IV Q 4-8h. *Child >1 y.o.-adult:* 5-10 mg IV.

Pediatric and Adult Drug Dosing

See index for generic names of proprietary meds

MEDICATION	PREPARATIONS	DOSING
Warfarin (Coumadin)	Tab: 2, 2.5, 5, 7.5, 10 mg	Dose varies with disease process and individual.
Zalcitabine (Hivid)	Tab: 0.375, 0.75 mg	Child >30 kg-adult: 0.75 mg Q 8h.
Zidovudine (Retrovir)	Liquid: 50 mg/5 ml Cap: 100 mg	Child <12 y.o.: 720 mg/m²/d divided Q 6h (max 200 mg/dose. See p. 165 for body surface area determination. Child >12 y.o.-adult: 500 mg/d po divided 200 mg-100 mg-200 mg on TID schedule.
Zolpidem tartrate (Ambien)	Tab: 5, 10 mg	Adult: 5-10 mg po at hs.

Prescription Eye Medications

Topical anesthetics (do not discharge patients on these meds)
Tetracaine *(Pontocaine)* HCl 0.5% .... 1-2 drops once only
Proparacaine *(Ophthaine)* HCl 0.5% .... 1-2 drops once only

Miotics (anti-glaucoma)
Pilocarpine 0.25-10% .... 1-2 drops Q 4-12h
Epinephrine 0.25-2% .... 1 drop Q 12h
Timolol 0.25-5% .... 1 drop Q 24h

Mydriatics (contraindicated in glaucoma)
A. Sympathomimetic
   Phenylephrine *(Mydfrin)* 0.12%, 2.5%, 10% .... 1-2 drops Q 6h
      Onset 30min, duration 12-24h, use cautiously if HTN present.
B. Anti-muscarinic
   Tropicamide *(Mydriacyl)* 0.5%, 1.0% .... 1-2 drops
      Max effect in 20-40min, duration 6-7h. 1% induces cycloplegia.
   Cyclopentolate *(Cyclogyl)* 1%, 2% .... 1 drop Q 5h x 2
      Max effect in 15-20min, duration 24h.
Homatropine 2%, 5%... 1-2 drops
   Onset 40min, max effect 3-4h, duration 24h.

Topical vasoconstrictors
Naphazoline HCl 0.012%,0.025% .... 1-2 drops Q 4h

Antibiotic solutions
Sodium sulfacetamide 10%, 15%, 30% .... 1-2 drops Q 2-3h
Gentamicin 0.3%.. 1-3 drops Q 2-3h
Ciprofloxacin (3.5 mg/ml)...................................... 1-2 drops Q 4-6h

Antibiotic ointments
Bacitracin, neomycin sulfate,
   polymixin sulfate ointment .... Apply Q 4h
Gentamicin 0.3%.. Apply Q 6h
Sodium sulfacetamide 10% .... Apply Q 6h

Prices of Oral Meds   *See index for generic names of proprietary meds*

Price to patient, based on a national survey of pharmacies. Quantities of medications in number of tabs or caps or in ml of liquid are those typically prescribed for each type of medication, for example, antibiotics, 1 week. Prices of generic drugs used unless only proprietary formulations available.

Drug - Quantity	Cost	Drug - Quantity	Cost
Acebutolol *Cap 200 mg* #30 ...	$30.42	Azithromycin *Cap 250 mg* #6	$55.59
Acebutolol *Cap 400 mg* #30	39.69	Beclomethasone *Inhaler* #1	33.12
Acetaminophen/codeine *A 120 mg,*		Benazepril *Tab 5 mg* #30	23.77
C 12 mg/5 ml 120 ml	9.09	Benazepril *Tab 40 mg* #30	23.77
Acetaminophen/codeine		Benztropine *Tab 1 mg* #12	5.42
Tab A 300 mg, C 30 mg #28	7.79	Benztropine *Tab 2 mg* #12	6.69
Acyclovir *Tab 800 mg* #28	103.75	Bepridil *Tab 200 mg* #30	77.55
Acyclovir *Cap 200 mg* #50	54.10	Bepridil *Tab 400 mg* #30	99.92
Acyclovir *200 mg/5ml* 250 ml	49.57	Betaxolol *Tab 10 mg* #30	27.16
Albuterol *Tab 2 mg* #90	21.64	Betaxolol *Tab 20 mg* #30	37.80
Albuterol *Tab SR 4 mg* #90	41.57	Bisacodyl *Tab 5 mg* #5	2.66
Albuterol *2 mg/5 ml* 600 ml	38.42	Bisacodyl *Supp 10 mg* #5	4.46
Aminophylline *Tab 200 mg*#120	10.03	Bisoprolol *Tab 5 mg* #30	25.98
Amlodipine *Tab 2.5 mg* #30	39.29	Bisoprolol *Tab 10 mg* #30	28.48
Amlodipine *Tab 5 mg* #30	39.66	Bitolterol *Inhaler* #1	27.50
Amlodipine *Tab 10 mg* #30	63.98	Bumetanide *Tab 0.5 mg* #30 ...	12.58
Amoxicillin *250 mg/5 ml* 100 ml	8.17	Bumetanide *Tab 1 mg* #30	16.05
Amoxicillin *Cap 250 mg* #21	6.31	Bumetanide *Tab 2 mg* #30	24.40
Amoxicillin *Cap 500 mg* #21	9.14	Butoconazole *Vag cream 2% with*	
Amoxicillin/clavulanate *A 250 mg,*		*applicator* #1	23.96
C 62.5 mg/5 ml 105 ml	47.32	Capsaicin *Cream 0.025%* 3 oz ..	20.66
Amoxicillin/clavulanate		Capsaicin *Cream 0.075%* 2 oz ..	31.18
Tab A 250, C 125 mg #21	49.17	Captopril *Tab 12.5 mg* #90	60.85
Amoxicillin/clavulanate		Captopril *Tab 25 mg* #90	62.87
Tab A 500 mg, C 125 mg #21	67.03	Captopril *Tab 37.5 mg* #90	114.00
Ampicillin *250/5 ml* 200 ml	9.44	Captopril *Tab 100 mg* #90	146.47
Ampicillin *Cap 250 mg* #28	7.00	Carbamazepine	
Ampicillin *Cap 500 mg* #28	8.25	*Tab 200 mg* #90	20.87
Astemizole *Tab 10 mg* #7	16.82	Carteolol *Tab 2.5 mg* #30	30.40
Atenolol *Tab 50 mg* #30	8.17	Carteolol *Tab 5 mg* #30	34.99
Atenolol *Tab 100 mg* #30	12.02	Cefaclor *250 mg/5ml* 150 ml ...	52.70

See index for generic names of proprietary meds **Prices of Oral Meds**

Drug - Quantity	Cost
Cefaclor *Cap 250 mg* #21	$48.11
Cefaclor *Cap 500 mg* #21	90.63
Cefadroxil *250 mg/5 ml* 100 ml	30.06
Cefadroxil *Cap 500 mg* #14	50.06
Cefadroxil *Tab 1 g* #14	83.77
Cefixime *100 mg/5ml* 100 ml ...	65.89
Cefixime *Tab 200 mg* #7	35.60
Cefixime *Tab 400 mg* #7	48.27
Cefpodoxime *100 mg/5 ml* 100 ml	62.06
Cefpodoxime *Tab 100 mg* #14 ...	29.44
Cefpodoxime *Tab 200 mg* #14 ...	50.14
Cefprozil *Tab 500 mg* #14	81.59
Cefuroxime *Tab 125 mg* #14	28.89
Cefuroxime *Tab 250 mg* #14	47.15
Cefuroxime *Tab 500 mg* #14	90.15
Cephalexin *250 mg/5ml* 200 ml	20.61
Cephalexin *Cap 250 mg* #28	12.40
Cephalexin *Cap 500 mg* #28	15.47
Cephalexin *Tab 250 mg* #28	25.87
Cephalexin *Tab 500 mg* #28	55.25
Cephradine *250 mg/5ml* 100 ml .	15.46
Cephradine *Cap 250 mg* #28	18.66
Cephradine *Cap 500 mg* #28	37.38
Chlorpropamide *Tab 250 mg* #30	5.81
Chlorthalidone *Tab 50 mg* #30	6.15
Cimetidine *Tab 300 mg* #120 ...	87.57
Cinoxacin *Cap 250 mg* #14	21.20
Cinoxacin *Cap 500 mg* #14	27.05
Ciprofloxacin *Tab 250 mg* #14 ..	40.52
Ciprofloxacin *Tab 500 mg* #14 ..	47.18
Cisapride *Tab 10 mg* #90	59.67
Clarithromycin *Tab 250 mg* #14	46.01
Clarithromycin *Tab 500 mg* #14	46.01
Clindamycin *Cap 150 mg* #28	27.85
Clonidine *Tab 0.1 mg* #60	7.43
Clonidine *Tab 0.2 mg* #60	9.72

Drug - Quantity	Cost
Clonidine *Tab 0.3 mg* #60	$11.90
Clonidine *Patch TTS-1* #4	32.35
Clonidine *Patch TTS-3* #4	72.83
Clotrimazole *1% cream* 45 g	16.59
Clotrimazole	
Oral troche 10 mg #70	57.09
Clotrimazole *Vag tab 100 mg* #7	13.67
Clotrimazole *Vag tab 500 mg* #1	18.04
Cloxacillin *125 mg/5ml* 200 ml	10.82
Cloxacillin *Cap 250 mg* #28	11.28
Cloxacillin *Cap 500 mg* #28	16.31
Codeine *15 mg/5 ml* 120 ml	8.98
Codeine *Tab 30 mg* #28	9.62
Colchicine *Tab 0.6 mg* #30	6.30
Cyclobenzaprine *Tab 10 mg* #21	15.21
Cyproheptadine *Tab 4 mg* #56 ..	7.79
Dicloxacillin	
62.5 mg/5 ml 200 ml	20.49
Dicloxacillin *Cap 250 mg* #28	14.66
Dicloxacillin *Cap 500 mg* #28	22.47
Diflunisal *Tab 250 mg* #14	16.61
Diflunisal *Tab 500 mg* #14	18.52
Diltiazem *Tab 30 mg* #90	29.93
Diltiazem *Tab 60 mg* #90	45.50
Diltiazem *Tab 90 mg* #90	63.09
Diltiazem *Tab 120 mg* #90	78.03
Diltiazem *Cap (Cardizem SR)*	
60 mg #60	44.61
Diltiazem *Cap (Cardizem SR)*	
90 mg #60	53.67
Diltiazem *Cap (Cardizem SR)*	
120 mg #60	67.86
Diltiazem *Cap (Cardizem CD)*	
120 mg #30	43.80
Diltiazem *Cap (Cardizem CD)*	
180 mg #30	41.55

Prices of Oral Meds   *See index for generic names of proprietary meds*

Drug - Quantity	Cost	Drug - Quantity	Cost
Diltiazem *Cap (Cardizem CD)* 240 mg #30	$54.89	Glyburide *Tab 5 mg* #30	$18.70
		Guanfacine *Tab 1 mg* #30	28.22
Diltiazem *Cap (Cardizem CD)* 300 mg #30	69.92	Guanfacine *Tab 2 mg* #30	36.20
Diltiazem *Cap (Dilacor XR)* 180 mg #30	36.12	Hydrochlorothiazide *Tab 50 mg* #30	4.62
Diltiazem *Cap (Dilacor XR)* 240 mg #30	36.57	Hydrochlorothiazide/spironolactone *Tab H 25, S 25 mg* #30	8.34
Diphenhydramine *Tab 50 mg* #28	5.19	Hydrochlorothiazide/spironolactone *Tab H 50, S 50 mg* #30	26.59
Diphenoxylate/atropine *D 2.5 mg, A 0.025 mg/5ml* 120 ml	14.23	Hydrochlorothiazide/triamterene *Cap H 25/T 50 mg* #30	12.50
Diphenoxylate/atropine *Tab D 2.5, A 0.025 mg* #28	5.35	Hydrocodone/acetaminophen *(Vicodin) H 5 mg, A 500 mg* #28	8.96
Docusate *Tab 100 mg* #60	4.34	Hydrocodone/acetaminophen *(Vicodin ES) H 7.5 mg, A 500 mg* #28	17.25
Doxazosin *Tab 1 mg* #30	31.18		
Doxazosin *Tab 8 mg* #30	33.90	Ibuprofen *100 mg/5ml* 120 ml.	10.49
Doxycycline *50 mg/ml* 60 ml	19.75	Ibuprofen *Tab 400 mg* #28	6.20
Doxycycline *Tab 100 mg* #14	8.53	Ibuprofen *Tab 800 mg* #28	7.43
Enalapril *Tab 2.5 mg* #60	47.07	Indapamide *Tab 2.5 mg* #30	24.64
Enalapril *Tab 10 mg* #60	59.40	Indomethacin *Cap 50 mg* #28	8.26
Enalapril *Tab 20 mg* #60	83.18	Ipratropium *Inhaler* #1	35.25
Erythromycin *Tab 250 mg* #28	7.86	Isosorbide dinitrate *(Isordil) Tab 10 mg* #120	8.27
Erythromycin *Tab 500 mg* #28	11.42	Isosorbide dinitrate *(Isordil) Tab 40 mg* #120	45.52
Erythromycin/sulfisoxazole *E 200 mg, S 600 mg/5 ml* 150 ml	16.20	Isradipine *Tab 2.5 mg* #60	36.23
Famciclovir *Tab 500 mg* #21	146.99	Isradipine *Tab 5 mg* #60	50.39
Famotidine *Tab 20 mg* #60	90.99	Ketorolac *Tab 10 mg* #28	37.47
Famotidine *Tab 40 mg* #60	169.83	Labetalol *Tab 100 mg* #60	29.97
Fluconazole *Tab 100 mg* #25	175.82	Labetalol *Tab 300 mg* #60	51.76
Fosinopril *Tab 10 mg* #30	26.44	Lindane *Lotion 1%* 1 oz	5.64
Fosinopril *Tab 20 mg* #30	28.25	Lisinopril *Tab 5 mg* #30	28.24
Furosemide *Tab 40 mg* #30	4.88	Lisinopril *Tab 40 mg* #30	43.12
Furosemide *Tab 80 mg* #30	5.85	Lomefloxacin *Tab 400 mg* #7	47.76
Glipizide *Tab 5 mg* #30	14.44	Loperamide *Cap 2 mg* #12	10.19
Glipizide *Tab 10 mg* #30	22.97		
Glyburide *Tab 1.25 mg* #30	9.04		

See index for generic names of proprietary meds **Prices of Oral Meds**

Drug - Quantity	Cost	Drug - Quantity	Cost
Loperamide *1 mg/5ml* 120 ml	$6.66	Nicardipine *SR Cap 60 mg* #60	$79.56
Loracarbef *100 mg/5ml* 100 ml	26.75	Nifedipine *Cap 10 mg* #90	25.77
Loracarbef *Cap 200 mg* #14	50.03	Nifedipine *Cap 20 mg* #90	57.57
Meclizine *Tab 25 mg* #21	5.31	Nifedipine *XL Cap 30 mg* #30	38.60
Meclizine *Tab 50 mg* #21	32.34	Nifedipine *XL Cap 60 mg* #30	63.23
Metaproterenol *Tab 10 mg* #120	26.23	Nifedipine *XL Cap 90 mg* #30	74.83
Metaproterenol *Tab 20 mg* #120	34.49	Nitroglycerin *SL tab 0.6 mg* #60	4.99
Metaproterenol *10 mg/5ml* 600 ml	24.36	Nitroglycerin *Tab 6.5 mg* #90	11.89
		Nitroglycerin *Tab 9 mg* #90	13.42
Metaproterenol *Inhaler* #1	18.00	Nitroglycerin *Transdermal patch 0.1 mg/h* #30	40.89
Metoclopramide *Tab 10 mg* #28	5.28	Nitroglycerin *Transdermal patch 0.6 mg/h* #30	47.59
Metoclopramide *5 mg/5ml* 120 ml	7.14	Nizatidine *Tab 150 mg* #60	94.07
Metolazone *Tab 2.5 mg* #30	16.96	Nizatidine *Tab 300 mg* #60	176.52
Metolazone *Tab 10 mg* #30	21.62	Norfloxacin *Tab 400 mg* #14	45.58
Metoprolol *Tab 50 mg* #60	29.03	Nystatin *Cream 100,000 U/g* 30 g	9.42
Metoprolol *Tab 100 mg* #60	41.43	Nystatin *Oral suspension 100,000 /ml* 100 ml	14.72
Metoprolol *XL Tab 50 mg* #30	16.78	Nystatin *Vag supp 100,000 U* #14	12.35
Metoprolol *XL Tab 100 mg* #30	21.34	Omeprazole *Tab 20 mg* #30	110.41
Metoprolol *XL Tab 200 mg* #30	42.70	Oxacillin *250 mg/5ml* 100 ml	8.61
Metronidazole *Tab 250 mg* #28	7.69	Oxacillin *Cap 250 mg* #28	11.07
Metronidazole *Tab 500 mg* #28	12.58	Oxacillin *Cap 500 mg* #28	17.03
Miconazole *Vag supp 100 mg* #7	14.02	Penicillin V *250 mg/5ml* 200 ml	8.34
Miconazole *Vag supp 200 mg* #3	26.85	Penicillin V *Cap 500 mg* #28	6.68
Nabumetone *Tab 500 mg* #14	18.60	Phenobarbital *Tab 32 mg* #30	4.65
Nabumetone *Tab 750 mg* #14	22.89	Phenytoin *Tab 100 mg* #90	19.35
Nadolol *Tab 40 mg* #30	30.06	Pindolol *Tab 5 mg* #60	44.13
Nadolol *Tab 120 mg* #30	52.57	Pindolol *Tab 10 mg* #60	55.86
Nadolol *Tab 160 mg* #30	58.60	Pirbuterol *Inhaler* #1	30.69
Naproxen *Tab 250 mg* #14	11.01	Piroxicam *Tab 10 mg* #14	19.91
Naproxen *Tab 500 mg* #14	15.98	Piroxicam *Tab 20 mg* #14	20.72
Nedocromil *Inhaler* #1	31.71	Prazosin *Cap 1 mg* #90	15.11
Nicardipine *Cap 20 mg* #90	40.05	Prazosin *Cap 5 mg* #90	29.15
Nicardipine *Cap 30 mg* #90	60.51	Prochlorperazine *Tab 5 mg* #28	22.00
Nicardipine *SR Cap 30 mg* #60	40.01		

Prices of Oral Meds *See index for generic names of proprietary meds*

Drug - Quantity	Cost	Drug - Quantity	Cost
Prochlorperazine *Tab 10 mg* #28	$30.72	Terbutaline *Tab 2.5 mg* #90	$27.59
Prochlorperazine *Supp 25 mg* #14	29.04	Terbutaline *Tab 5 mg* #90	38.34
Propoxyphene/acetaminophen (Darvocet-N 50)		Terbutaline *Inhaler* #1	25.48
P 50, A 325 mg #28	11.46	Terconazole *Vag cream 0.4%* 45 g tube with applicator #7	27.84
Propoxyphene/acetaminophen (Darvocet-N 100)		Terconazole *Vag cream 0.8%* 45 g tube with applicator #3	28.44
P 100, A 650 mg #28	8.69	Terconazole *Vag supp 80 mg* #3	28.50
Propranolol *Tab 80 mg* #30	10.86	Terfenadine *Tab 60 mg* #14	16.89
Propranolol *SR Cap 80 mg* #30	23.59	Tetracycline *Cap 500 mg* #28	6.05
Propranolol *SR Cap 160 mg* #30	39.19	Timolol *Tab 5 mg* #60	22.74
Pseudoephedrine *30 mg/5ml* 120 ml	5.59	Timolol *Tab 10 mg* #60	29.96
Pseudoephedrine *Tab 60 mg* #28	4.32	Timolol *Tab 20 mg* #60	51.37
Quinapril *Tab 5 mg* #30	31.64	Tioconazole *Vag ointment 6.5%* 4.6 g with applicator #1	27.69
Quinapril *Tab 10 mg* #30	31.64	Triamcinolone *Inhaler* #1	46.18
Quinapril *Tab 40 mg* #30	31.64	Trimethobenzamide *Cap 100 mg* #21	13.58
Ramipril *Tab 1.25 mg* #30	22.67	Trimethobenzamide *Cap 250 mg* #21	12.84
Ramipril *Tab 10 mg* #30	31.18	Trimethoprim *Tab 100 mg* #14	7.43
Ranitidine *Tab 150 mg* #60	95.10	Trimethoprim *Tab 200 mg* #14	11.12
Ranitidine *Tab 300 mg* #60	168.59	Trimethoprim/sulfa *T 40, S 200 mg/5ml* 120 ml	6.92
Scopolamine *Transderm patch 1.5 mg* #4	20.99	Trimethoprim/sulfa (SS) *Tab T 80, S 400 mg* #14	6.03
Silver sulfadiazine *Cream 1%* 25 g	8.26	Trimethoprim/sulfa (DS) *Tab T 160, S 800 mg* #14	7.11
Silver sulfadiazine *Cream 1%* 50 g	9.39	Verapamil *Tab 40 mg* #90	26.75
Silver sulfadiazine *Cream 1%* 400 g	28.79	Verapamil *Tab 80 mg* #90	18.43
Spironolactone *Tab 25 mg* #120	11.17	Verapamil *Tab 120 mg* #90	17.00
Spironolactone *Tab 50 mg* #120	83.71	Verapamil *SR Tab 120 mg* #30	27.30
Spironolactone *Tab 100 mg* #120	136.76	Verapamil *SR Tab 180 mg* #30	34.21
Sucralfate *Tabs 1 g* #120	86.12	Verapamil *SR Tab 240 mg* #30	37.62
Sulfamethoxazole *Tab 1 g* #14	8.39	Zidovudine *Cap 100 mg* #90	139.03
Sulfisoxazole *Tab 500 mg* #28	7.90	Zidovudine *50 mg/5ml* 480 ml	77.83
Sulindac *Tab 150 mg* #28	16.82		
Sulindac *Tab 200 mg* #28	19.13		

Dental Anatomy

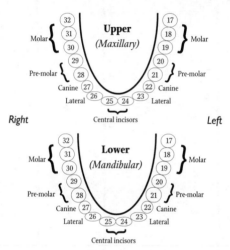

Hand Sensory Nerve Innervation

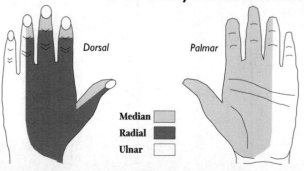

Hand Motor Exam

Nerve = nerve innervation
M = median; U = ulnar; R = radial

Extrinsic Hand Flexors

Muscle(s)	Nerve	Test
Flexor pollicis longus	M	Flexion of the distal phalanx of the thumb.
Flexor digitorum profundus	MU*	Test 2nd to 5th separately. MCP and PIP of tested finger held in extension by examiner while pt flexes DIP joint.
Flexor digitorum superficialis	M	Test 2nd to 5th separately. Untested fingers are held in extension by examiner while patient flexes PIP joint.
Flexor carpi radialis	M	While the patient, making a fist, flexes the wrist against
Palmaris longus	M	resistance, these tendons are palpated respectively in the
Flexor carpi ulnaris	U	radial, central, and ulnar regions of the volar wrist.

* Thumb and index fingers by median; ring and little fingers by ulnar

Extrinsic Hand Extensors

Dorsal wrist compartment/muscle(s)	Nerve	Test
1 Abductor pollicis longus	R	With all fingers extended, patient abducts thumb, keeping
Extensor pollicis brevis	R	it in the plane of the other fingers.
2 Extensor carpi radialis longus	R	Clenching a fist, the patient extends at the wrist against
Extensor carpi radialis brevis	R	resistance. Tendons palpable over dorsoradial wrist.
3 Extensor pollicis longus	R	Hand palm-down on table, patient lifts thumb straight up.

4	*Extensor digitorum communis* *Extensor indicis proprius*	R R	Extension simultaneously of second through fifth fingers, examiner noting MCP extension. Test EIP separately by extension of index finger from a clenched fist, noting MCP extension.
5	*Extensor digiti minimi*	R	After making a fist, the little finger is extended. Examiner notes extension at MCP joint.
6	*Extensor carpi ulnaris*	R	Patient extends wrist and deviates it to the ulnar side. Tendon palpable over dorsal wrist distal to ulnar head.

Intrinsic Hand Muscles

GROUP	MUSCLE(S)	NERVE	TEST
Thenar	*Abductor pollicis brevis* *Opponens pollicis* *Flexor pollicis brevis*	M M MU*	Patient touches thumb to little finger keeping nails parallel.
	Adductor pollicis	U	Patient forcibly holds paper between thumb and radial side of the index proximal phalanx.
	Interosseous *Lumbricals*	U MU†	Holding hand palm down, patient spreads fingers.
Hypothenar	*Abductor digiti minimi* *Flexor digiti minimi* *Opponens digiti minimi*	U U U	Holding hand palm down, and starting with fingers pressed together, the patient moves the little finger away from the others.

* Shared by median and ulnar   † Index and middle by median; ring and little fingers by ulnar

Hand Muscles by Nerve Innervation

Median

Flexor carpi radialis
Palmaris longus
Flexor digitorum superficialis
Flexor digitorum profundus
    (thumb, index, and usually long fingers)
Flexor pollicis longus
Abductor pollicis brevis
Flexor pollicis brevis (shared with ulnar)
Opponens pollicis
Lumbricals (index and long fingers)

Radial

Extensor carpi radialis longus and *brevis*
Extensor digitorum communis
Extensor digiti minimi
Extensor carpi ulnaris
Abductor pollicis longus
Extensor pollicis longus and *brevis*
Extensor indicis proprius

Ulnar

Flexor carpi ulnaris
Flexor digitorum profundus
    (ring, little, and sometimes long finger)
Adductor pollicis
Flexor pollicis brevis (shared with median)
Abductor, opponens, and *flexor digiti minimi*
Lumbricals (little and ring fingers)
Interossei

Spinal Cord Levels Sensory and Motor

Sensory		Motor	
C2	Occiput	C1-C4	Flexion, extension, rotation of neck
C3	Thyroid cartilage	C3-C5	Spontaneous breathing
C4	Suprasternal notch	C3-C5	Shrugging of shoulders
C5	Below clavicle	C5-C6	Elbow flexion
C6	Thumb	C6-C8	Elbow extension
C7	Index finger	C6-C8	Hand extension
C8	Small finger	C6-C8	Finger extension
T4	Nipple line	C7-T1	Hand flexion
T10	Umbilicus	C7-T1	Finger flexion
L1	Inguinal ligament	L1-L3	Hip flexion
L2-L3	Medial thigh	L2-L4	Leg extension
L4	Knee	L3-L4	Hip adduction
L5	Lateral calf	L4-S2	Hip abduction
S1	Lateral foot	L4-S1	Foot dorsiflexion
S2-S4	Perineum	L5-S2	Foot plantar flexion
S2	Gluteus maximus	L5-S1	Toe extension
S3-4	Anal sphincter	L5-S2	Toe flexion
		S2-S4	Sphincter tone

Reflexes			
CN VII	Corneal	L2-L4	Patellar
CN IX	Gag	S1	Achilles
C5-C6	Biceps	S1-S2	Plantar
C6-C7	Triceps	S2-S4	Bulbocavernosus
T1-T2	Ciliospinal	S4-S5	Anal
L1	Cremasteric		

Sensory Dermatomes

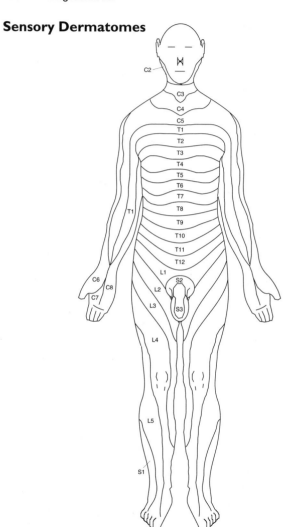

Sensory Dermatomes

Posterior

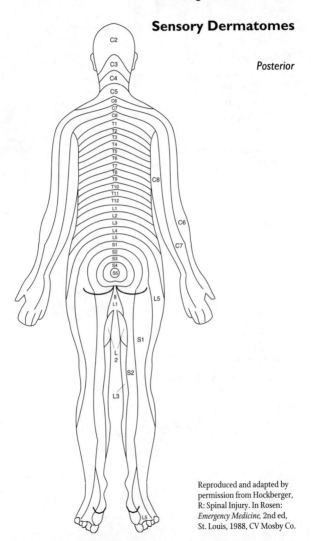

Reproduced and adapted by
permission from Hockberger,
R: Spinal Injury. In Rosen:
Emergency Medicine, 2nd ed,
St. Louis, 1988, CV Mosby Co.

Cervical Spine Radiologic Parameters

In lateral view:

Atlanto-dental interval = distance from anterior aspect of odontoid to posterior aspect of C1 (**a**). Normal = 0-3 mm (children 0-4.5 mm). In adults 3-7 mm indicates rupture of transverse ligament. > 7mm indicates rupture of alar and apical dentate ligaments.

If the anterior height of any vertebral body (**b1**) is greater by more than 3 mm than the posterior height (**b2**), a vertebral body fracture is likely.

Soft tissue from anterior aspect of each vertebral body to tracheal air space should measure not more than the following:

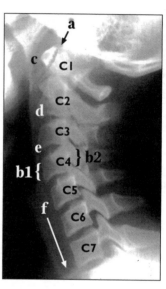

- At C1 (**c**), 10 mm.
- At the bottom of C2 (**d**), 5 mm.
- At the bottom of C3 (**e**), 7 mm.
- From the bottom of C5 to the bottom of C7 (**f**), 20 mm.

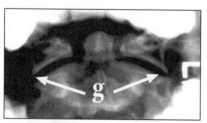

Concept and research courtesy of Steve Yucht, M.D.

In AP odontoid view:

In AP view, sum of overhang of both facets of C1 on C2 > 7 mm = rupture of transverse ligament (**g**).

Cervical Spine Injuries: Stable and Unstable

Flexion

Wedge fracture .... *Stable*

Clay-shoveler's fracture .... *Stable*

Subluxation... *Potentially unstable*

Bilateral facet dislocation .... *Unstable*

Flexion teardrop .... *Unstable*

Atlantooccipital dislocation .... *Unstable*

Anterior atlantoaxial dislocation
    with or without fracture .... *Unstable*

Odontoid fracture with lateral
    displacement... *Unstable*

Fracture of transverse process............................. *Stable*

Extension

Posterior neural arch fracture C1 .... *Stable*

Hangman's fracture C2 .... *Unstable*

Extension teardrop fracture .... *Unstable in extension;
                                                                        stable in flexion*

Posterior atlantoaxial dislocation
    with or without fracture .... *Unstable*

Vertical compression

Burst fracture .... *Stable*

Jefferson fracture C1.. *Unstable*

Fractures of articular pillar
    and vertebral body .... *Stable*

Rotation

Unilateral facet dislocation .... *Stable*

Rotary atlantoaxial dislocation .... *Unstable*

Coma: Correlating Exam Findings with Level of Brain Dysfunction

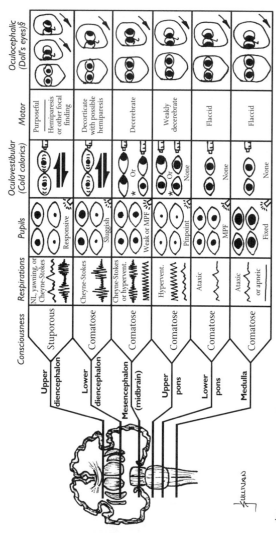

* Dysconjugate response indicates structural brainstem lesion. MPF = mid-position fixed.
§ Doll's eye testing contraindicated in patients with suspected cervical spine injury.

Toxicology

General Protocol for Ingestions

I. **Gastrointestinal decontamination**

A. *Ipecac* 30 ml po for children >12 y.o. and adults, 15 ml po for ambulatory children, or *gastric lavage* is indicated if either can be initiated within 2h of the ingestion. Never administer ipecac if the toxic agent is associated with CNS and/or cardiovascular depression, or is corrosive, or if gag reflex is absent. *Intubation* prior to gastric lavage should be considered in patients with absent gag reflex, or for those who have ingested a toxic product with a hydrocarbon carrier (e.g., pesticides). Consider decontamination more than 2h after ingestion if the patient is critically ill, the substance ingested causes pylorospasm, or if the substance ingested is a seed (e.g., jimson weed).

B. *Activated charcoal* 1 g/kg should be administered to all patients except those with caustic or hydrocarbon ingestions.

C. *Whole gut lavage using polyethylene glycol* containing solutions is recommended for drugs not bound to activated charcoal (e.g. lithium or iron), for massive ingestions, body packers, or sustained release/enteric coated formulations. Dose: 1-2 l/h in adults, 40 ml/kg/h in children until rectal effluent is clear. Contraindicated if an ileus is present.

D. *Cathartics* should be administered initially and then once every 24h. *Sorbitol* 1 g/kg is most effective but must not be given if an ileus is present or if aspiration is possible.

E. *Multiple dose activated charcoal* 0.5 g/kg Q 2-4h with one dose of cathartic/day is indicated for theophylline, phenobarbital, salicylates, carbamazepine, phenytoin, mushrooms containing amatoxins, digitoxin, and enteric coated or sustained release formulations.

General Protocol for Toxic Ingestion

II. Observation

All patients with alleged ingestion must be closely observed for at least 6h. When in doubt as to the nature of the ingestion, administer activated charcoal and observe. Remember: a negative drug screen does not rule out ingestion of a toxic agent. The following substances require prolonged observation (18-24h):

A. oral hypoglycemic agents
B. lithium
C. phenytoin
D. *Lomotil* (diphenoxylate/atropine)
E. monoamine oxidase inhibitors
F. colchicine
G. sustained release/enteric coated preparations

Protocol for Cutaneous Decontamination

Hospital personnel must don appropriate protective equipment prior to patient decontamination. Proceed in a stepwise fashion, moving to the next step if the previous one has been unsuccessful:

A. warm water irrigation (exception: elemental metals explode on contact with water)
B. gentle soaps
C. 50% detergent/50% corn meal
D. dilute bleach
E. Specific cutaneous antidotes:
1. phenol—mineral oil/isopropanol/polyethylene glycol solution.
2. chromium—topical and systemic ascorbic acid/topical EDTA.
3. phosphorus—Woods lamp for detection/ignites on contact with air (keep covered with oils).
4. hydrofluoric acid—topical 2.5% calcium gluconate gel until pain relief obtained. For intractable pain:
   a. hand injuries—infuse calcium gluconate 10% 10 ml in 40 ml normal saline via radial arterial line over 4h while on cardiac monitor.
   b. all other areas—inject calcium gluconate 10% 0.5 ml/sq cm of involved skin.

Protocol for Tricyclic Antidepressant Ingestions

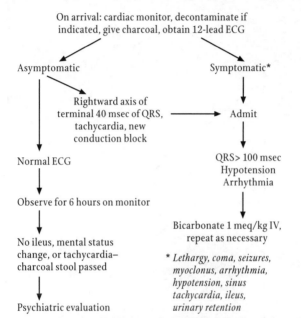

On arrival: cardiac monitor, decontaminate if indicated, give charcoal, obtain 12-lead ECG

Asymptomatic

Symptomatic*

Rightward axis of terminal 40 msec of QRS, tachycardia, new conduction block → Admit

Normal ECG

Observe for 6 hours on monitor

No ileus, mental status change, or tachycardia–charcoal stool passed

Psychiatric evaluation

QRS> 100 msec
Hypotension
Arrhythmia

Bicarbonate 1 meq/kg IV, repeat as necessary

* *Lethargy, coma, seizures, myoclonus, arrhythmia, hypotension, sinus tachycardia, ileus, urinary retention*

Osmolality Formulae

Calculated osmolality (mOsm/kg) = $2Na + BUN / 2.8 + Glucose / 18$

If measured osmolality (by freezing point depression) is more than ten greater than calculated osmolality, unmeasured osmoles should be presumed to be present. However, a normal "gap" does not rule out the presence of toxic alcohols.

Osmol ratios: to calculate contribution to measured osmolality in mosm/kg, divide concentration in mg/dl by these numbers:

Ethylene glycol	*Isopropanol*	*Ethanol*	*Methanol*
6.2	6.0	4.6	3.2

Salicylate Overdose Nomogram

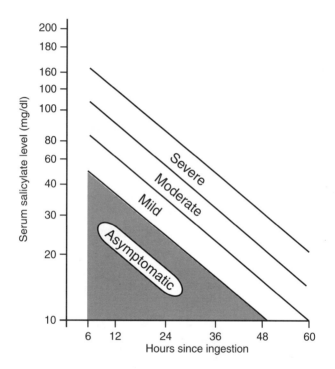

The Done nomogram for estimating severity of salicylate overdose, based on time since ingestion and level on presentation. This nomogram is only reliable for a single acute ingestion (not for chronic intoxication, or when ingestion is of enteric coated or liquid preparations, or in patients with abnormal volume status or pH).

Reproduced by permission of *Pediatrics* 1968; 41:106.

Acetaminophen Overdose Nomogram

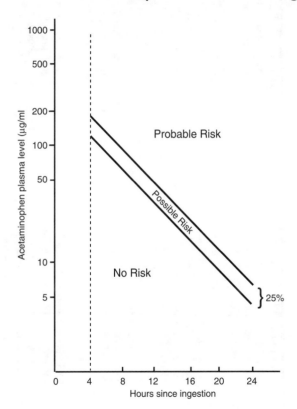

For evaluating need for treatment with N-acetylcysteine, based on time since a single, acute ingestion and plasma concentration on presentation. Treatment should be considered when levels fall above the area of "no risk." Determinations prior to four hours may not represent peak levels.

Reproduced with permission, *Arch Int Med* 1981; 141:380-385. Copyright AMA.

Toxidromes

DRUG	SYMPTOMS/SIGNS	MANAGEMENT PRINCIPLES
Sympathomimetics (*Cocaine, amphetamines*)	Tachycardia, tachypnea, mydriasis, hyperthermia, altered mentation, coma, agitation, seizure, rhabdomyolysis.	Benzodiazepines IV for agitation, aggressive cooling, short-acting cardiovascular agents, benzodiazepines and barbiturates for seizures, measures to correct acidosis.
Anticholinergics (*Antihistamines, over the counter sleep aids, anti-psychotics, plants and mushrooms*)	*Central:* altered mentation, coma, agitation, seizure, hyperthermia. *Peripheral:* tachycardia, ileus, urinary retention, mydriasis, dry skin and mucous membranes.	Same as for sympathomimetics. Physostigmine only for intractable seizures or supraventricular tachycardia with hemodynamic instability. Dose 0.5 mg over 5min (*child*) or 1-2 mg IV over 5min (*adult*).
Cholinergics (*Organophosphates, carbamates*)	Vomiting, diarrhea, salivation, lacrimation, bronchorrhea, fasciculations, paralysis.	Aggressive airway management and pulmonary toilet. For organophosphates/carbamates: atropine *and* pralidoxime—for dosing see p. 129, 131. *Worsening of carbaryl OD reported with pralidoxime—avoid.*
Opiates	CNS and respiratory depression, miosis, hypothermia. Meperidine may cause myoclonus/seizures. Propoxyphene may cause seizures and cardiac conduction blocks.	Naloxone —for dosing see p. 131. Drugs which may require higher doses of naloxone than other narcotics: methadone, pentazocine, propoxyphene, diphenoxylate, fentanyl.

Treatable by Hemodialysis or Hemoperfusion

HD = hemodialysis; HP = hemoperfusion

Substance	Method of choice	Indication
Ethylene glycol	HD	Altered mentation, hemodynamic instability, renal failure, metabolic acidosis, serum level > 25 mg/dl. *Add for children:* measured osmolality >380 mosm/l.
Isopropanol	HD	Hypotension, coma, level >400 mg/dl.
Lithium	HD	Significant clinical symptoms, serum level >4 mmol/l (less if intoxication chronic).
Methanol	HD	Visual changes, altered mentation, metabolic acidosis, serum level >25 mg/dl.
Salicylate	HD	Significant clinical symptoms: pulmonary edema, any neurologic sx, renal failure, worsening condition despite alkalinization, inability to alkalinize urine, metabolic acidosis, acute serum level approaching 100 mg/dl, chronic serum level approaching 40-60 mg/dl.
Theophylline	HP	Significant symptoms, seizures, acute serum levels approaching 100 µg/ml or chronic levels approaching 40-60 µg/ml.

Antidotes to Specific Overdoses

Overdose	Antidote	Initial Dose
Acetaminophen	N-acetylcysteine (*Mucomyst*)	*Child/adult:* 140 mg/kg po initial dose, then 70 mg/kg po Q4h for 17 doses.
Benzodiazepines	Flumazenil *See also p. 63*	*Child/adult:* for reversal of CNS depression from overdose (*not for mixed ingestions or in pts who are chronically benzodiazepine dependent or in those with elevated ICP*): 0.2 mg IV over 30sec. If no effect, try 0.3 mg IV over 30sec. If still no effect, try 0.5 mg IV over 30sec, then repeat Q 1min until total 3 mg given.
Beta-blockers	Glucagon *and/or*	*Child:* 50 μg/kg IV over 1min. *Adult:* 5-10 mg IV over 1min. *Not with phenol diluent for these large doses.*
	Atropine *and/or* Epinephrine	*Child/adult:* 0.01 mg/kg IV. *Child/adult:* start 0.1 μg/kg/min infusion, titrate to desired effect.
Botulism	Trivalent anti-toxin	*Child/adult:* 1-2 vials.
Calcium channel blockers	Calcium chloride 10% *and/or*	*Child:* 20 mg (0.2 ml)/kg IV over 5min. *Adult:* 1 g (10 ml) IV over 5min. Give slowly while on a cardiac monitor.

	Glucagon *and/or*	*Child:* 50 µg/kg IV over 1min. *Adult:* 5-10 mg IV over 1min. *Not with phenol diluent at these large doses.*
	Beta/alpha adrenergic agonists	As needed.
Carbamates	Atropine	*Child:* 0.02 mg/kg IV initial dose. *Adult:* 2 mg IV initial dose. May require larger doses. Dosing as for organophosphates.
	Pralidoxime	
Carbon disulfide	Pyridoxine (Vitamin B6)	*Child/adult:* 70 mg/kg IV over 15-30min.
Coumarin compounds	Vitamin K1 *and/or*	*Child <1 y.o.:* 1 mg in 20-50 ml IV Q 4-8h. *Child >1 y.o.-adult:* 5-10 mg IV at 1 mg/min.
	Fresh frozen plasma	Dose variable.
Cyanide	Amyl nitrite perles *and* Sodium nitrite 3% *and* Sodium thiosulfate 25% *and* 100% 02	*Child/adult:* inhale 30 sec/min in 02 mask. *Child/adult:* 0.33 ml/kg IV over 5min (max 10 ml). *Child/adult:* 1.65 ml/kg IV over 10min (max 50 ml). *Child/adult:* concomitant with above.
Cyclic antidepressants	Sodium bicarbonate	*Child/adult:* if QRS > 100 msec, hypotension, or arrhythmia: initial dose 1 mEq/kg IV, then repeat boluses to maintain serum pH > 7.5.

Antidotes to Specific Overdoses

Overdose	Antidote	Initial Dose
Digitalis	Digoxin-specific antibody fragments	*Child/adult:* calculate digoxin load by *either* 1) # pills x mg/pill x 0.7, *or* 2) .0056 x wt in kg x serum dig. level in ng/l. Digoxin load/0.6 = IV dose in # vials needed. If hemodynam. unstable, give 10-20 vials (40 mg/vial) IV *(child/adult).*
Ethylene glycol	Ethanol 10% in D5W *and* Pyridoxine *and* Thiamine	*Child/adult:* 10 ml/kg over 1h, then infuse 1 ml/kg/h to target level of 100 mg/dl. *Child/adult:* 50 mg IV Q6h. *Child:* 50 mg IV. *Adult:* 100 mg IV.
***Gyromitra* esculenta mushrooms**	Pyridoxine (Vitamin B6)	*Child/adult:* 25 mg/kg IV over 15-30min.
Heparin	Protamine sulfate	*Child/adult:* 1 mg IV/100 U heparin given.
Iron	Deferoxamine	*Child/adult:* for prolonged GI sx, lethargy, level >500 mg/dl: 15 mg/kg/h infusion.
Isoniazid	Pyridoxine (Vitamin B6)	*Child:* 70 mg/kg IV. *Adult:* 1 mg IV for each mg of INH ingested, max 5 g.
Methanol	Ethanol 10% in D5W *and* Leucovorin	*Child/adult:* 10 ml/kg over 1h, then infuse 1 ml/kg/h to target level of 100 mg/dl. *Child/adult:* 1-2 mg/kg IV Q4-6h.

Methemoglobinemia	Methylene blue	*Child/adult:* for symptoms or if MetHg >30%: 1-2 mg/kg.
Opiates	Naloxone	*Child <20 kg:* 0.1 mg/kg IV. *Child >20 kg-adult:* 2 mg IV. Repeat to max 10 mg. *Infusion:* give ²⁄₃ of that initially needed to awaken patient per hour IV.
Organophosphates	Atropine *and*	*Child:* 0.02 mg/kg/dose IV. *Adult:* 2 mg/dose IV. *Repeat as necessary to dry secretions.*
	Pralidoxime	*Child:* 25-40 mg/kg IV over 10min, max 1 g; repeat Q 6-12h. *Adult:* 1 g IV over 10min, then 500 mg/h infusion.
Phenothiazines *(Dystonic reaction only)*	Diphenhydramine *or* Benztropine mesylate	*Child/adult:* 1-2 mg/kg IV slowly. *Adult:* 25-50 mg IM/IV. *Adult (only):* 1-2 mg IM/IV.
Quinidine Quinine Tricyclic antidepressants Type IA/IC antiarrythmics	Sodium bicarbonate	*Child/adult:* if QRS >100 msec, hypotension, or arrhythmia: initial dose 1 mEq/kg IV, then repeat boluses to maintain serum pH >7.5.

Phone Resources for Toxicologic Information

Acute poisoning
Your Regional Poison Control Center phone .... _____
If none available, Children's Hospital of Michigan
Regional Poison Control Center, Detroit, MI
24 hours a day... *in Michigan* 1-(800) POISON-1
outside Michigan (313) 745-5711

Toxic waste disposal
Environmental Protection Agency, Public Information Center,
401 M Street S.W., Washington, D.C. 20460
9 a.m.–4:30 p.m. Eastern M-F... (202) 260-2080

Hazardous spill containment
CHEMTREC, 2501 M Street N.W., Washington, D.C. 20037
24 hours a day.. (800) 424-9300

Pesticides
National Pesticide Network, Texas Tech University Health Sciences
Center, Thompson Hall, Room S129, Lubbock, Texas 79430
8 a.m.–6 p.m. Central M-F .... (800) 858-7378

Hazardous chemical reports
National Response Center, U.S. Coast Guard Headquarters,
Attention: FOIA G-TPS-2, Room 2611, 2100 Second St. S.W.,
Washington, D.C. 20593
24 hours a day.. (800) 424-8802

Identification of unknown chemicals
American Chemical Society, 1120 Vermont Ave. N.W.,
Washington D.C. 20005
8:30 a.m.–5 p.m. Eastern M-F.. (800) 227-5558

Contaminated food/drugs
Food & Drug Administration, 5600 Fishers La., Rockville, MD 20857
Drugs: *8 a.m.–4:30 p.m. Eastern M-F* .... (301) 594-1012
Food: *24 hours a day* .... (301) 443-1240

Drugs, chemicals, and radiation in pregnancy
Motherisk, Division of Clinical Pharmacology, Hospital for Sick
Children, 555 University Ave., Toronto Ontario M5GlX8
9 a.m.–5 p.m. Eastern M-F.. (416) 598-6780

4
Trauma

Tetanus Wound Prophylaxis

Number of previous TD doses	Tetanus-prone wounds (see #4 below)		Non-tetanus prone wounds	
	Toxoid	TIG	Toxoid	TIG
Not known	Yes	Yes	Yes	No
0-1	Yes	Yes	Yes	No
2	Yes	No*	Yes	No
≥3	No#	No	No†	No

* Yes if wound more than 24 hours old
# Yes if more than 5 years since last dose
† Yes if more than 10 years since last dose

Note:
1) For children less than 7 y.o., Diphtheria-Tetanus-Pertussis (DPT) is preferred unless pertussis is contraindicated; all others should receive Diphtheria-Tetanus (TD). *See pediatric imunization schedule p. 175.*
2) TIG = tetanus immune globulin. Dose is 250-500 U IM for both children and adults.
3) When TIG and TD are given concurrently, use separate syringes and inject at separate sites.
4) Tetanus-prone wounds are suggested by:
   - More than 12 hours since injury
   - Blunt mechanism of injury
   - Signs of infection present
   - Devitalized or ischemic tissue present
   - Contaminants—soil, feces, saliva—in wound

Revised Adult Trauma Score *(Pediatric trauma score, p. 136)*

CRITERION		SCORE
Respiratory rate	10 - 24	**4**
	25 - 35	**3**
	≥ 36	**2**
	1 - 9	**1**
	0	**0**
Systolic blood pressure	≥ 90	**4**
	76 - 89	**3**
	50 - 75	**2**
	1 - 49	**1**
	0 (no pulse)	**0**
Glasgow Coma Scale	*See facing page*	
Coma scale points:	13 - 15	**4**
	9 - 12	**3**
	6 - 8	**2**
	4 - 5	**1**
	3	**0**

Probability of Survival by Overall Revised Trauma Score

12	0.995	**8**	0.667	**4**	0.333
11	0.969	**7**	0.636	**3**	0.333
10	0.879	**6**	0.630	**2**	0.286
9	0.766	**5**	0.455	**1**	0.250
				0	0.037

From *J Trauma* 1989; 29:623.

(Pediatric coma scale, p. 137)   **Adult Glasgow Coma Scale**

CRITERION	SCORE

Eye opening response

Spontaneous—already open with blinking **4**
To speech—not necessary to request eye opening **3**
To pain—stimulus should not be to the face **2**
None—make note if eyes are swollen shut **1**

Verbal response

Oriented—knows name, age, etc. **5**
Confused conversation—still answers questions **4**
Inappropriate words—speech is either
    exclamatory or at random **3**
Incomprehensible sounds—do not confuse with
    partial respiratory obstruction **2**
None—make note if patient is intubated **1**

Best upper limb motor response (pain applied to nailbed)

Obeys—moves limb to command; pain is not required **6**
Localizes—changing the location of the painful
    stimulus causes the limb to follow **5**
Withdraws—pulls away from painful stimulus **4**
Abnormal flexion—decorticate posturing **3**
Extensor response—decerebrate posturing **2**
No response **1**

Pediatric Trauma Score

Patients with an overall score of < 8 should be triaged to a Pediatric Trauma Center.

	Score		
	+ 2	**1**	**- 1**
Weight	> 20 kg	10-20 kg	< 10 kg
Airway	Normal	Oral or nasal airway	Intubation or cricothyroidotomy
Blood pressure	> 90 mm Hg	50 - 90 mm Hg	< 50 mm Hg
Level of consciousness	Awake and alert	Obtunded or any LOC	Comatose
Open wound	None	Minor	Major or penetrating
Fractures	None	Single simple	Open or multiple

Probability of Survival by Overall Pediatric Trauma Score

12 .... 1.00	**6** 0.92	**0** 0.26
10 .... 1.00	**4** 0.68	**-2** 0.08
8 .... 0.98	**2** 0.60	**-4** 0.00

From *J Pediatr Surg* 1987; 22:14.

Pediatric Coma Scale

	Score	*Infants*	*Children*
Eye	4	Spontaneous	Spontaneous
opening	3	To speech or sound	To speech
	2	To painful stimuli	To pain
	1	None	None
Verbal	5	Coos, babbles	Oriented
response	4	Irritable cry, consolable	Confused
	3	Cries to pain	Inappropriate words
	2	Moans to pain	Incomprehensible words
	1	None	None
Motor	6	Spontaneous movement	Obeys commands
response	5	Localizes pain	Localizes pain
	4	Withdraws to pain	Withdraws to pain
	3	Flexes — decorticate	Flexes — decorticate
	2	Extends — decerebrate	Extends — decerebrate
	1	None	None

Burn Surface Area

Adult Burn Surface Area

"Rule of nines"

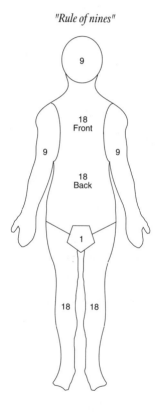

1% of body area = approximately area of patient's palmar hand surface

Burn Surface Area

Pediatric Burn Surface Area

Body area	AGE IN YEARS			
	0–1	1–4	4–9	10–15
Head	19	17	13	10
Neck	2	2	2	2
Chest or back (each)	13	13	13	13
Buttock (each)	2.5	2.5	2.5	2.5
Genitalia	1	1	1	1
Upper arm (each)	4	4	4	4
Lower arm (each)	3	3	3	3
Hand (each)	2.5	2.5	2.5	2.5
Thigh (each)	5.5	6.5	8.5	8.5
Lower leg (each)	5	5	5	6
Foot (each)	3.5	3.5	3.5	3.5

Indications for Admission

- Partial thickness > 20% or full thickness > 10%.
- Burns of hands, face, eyes, ears, feet, or perineum.
- Inhalation injury, electrical burns, or associated serious trauma.
- High risk patient, i.e., diabetes, obesity, liver disease, suspected child abuse.

Fluid Management

Ringer's lactate 2-4 ml/kg /% of body surface area over the first 24 hours with half over the first 8 hours and the remainder over the ensuing 16 hours, calculated from the time the burn is sustained. Add maintenance fluids for infants. This formula is meant as a guide — fluid management should be adjusted in accordance with clinical signs.

Tetanus prophylaxis

Adequacy of tetanus immunization should be ascertained, and toxoid and immune globulin administered when indicated (p. 133).

Rabies Prophylaxis

Geographic Area	Animals	Treatment Recommendation	
		Bite	*Non-bite Contact§*
Group 1: rabies endemic or suspected in species involved in the exposure	Bats anywhere in the U.S.; raccoons, skunks, foxes; mongooses in Puerto Rico; dogs in most developing countries and in the U.S. along Mexican border (3-80% rabid)	*Treat**	*Treat**
Group 2: rabies not endemic in species involved in the exposure, but endemic in other terrestrial animals in area	Most wild carnivores (wolves, bobcats, bears) and groundhogs (2-20% rabid)	*Treat**	*Treat* or consult†*
	Dogs and cats (0.1-2% rabid)	*Observe¶ or consult†*	*Observe¶ or consult†*
	Rodents and lagomorphs except groundhogs (about 0.01% rabid)	*Consult† or do not treat*	*Do not treat*
Group 3: rabies not endemic in species involved in the exposure or in other terrestrial animals in area	Dogs, cats, many wild terrestrial animals in Washington, Idaho, Utah, Nevada, Colorado (0.01-0.1% rabid)	*Consult† or do not treat*	*Consult† or do not treat*

§ Rabies develops in 5-60% if bitten, 0.1-0.2% if scratched or licked in open wound or mucous membrane.

* Treat = treatment with rabies immune globulin (RIG) and rabies vaccine—see p. 27 for treatment details.

† Consult = with state/local health dept. If rabies risk low and animal's brain available, Rx sometimes delayed up to 48h.

¶ Observe = After bite from domestic dog/cat, confine animal for 10d; if signs of rabies occur, treat immediately. After bite from stray or unwanted dog/cat, animal should be killed and head shipped to qualified lab for exam.

By permission of *N Engl J Med* 1993; 329:1635.

5
Critical Care

ACLS Protocols

Ventricular Fibrillation/Pulseless Ventricular Tachycardia

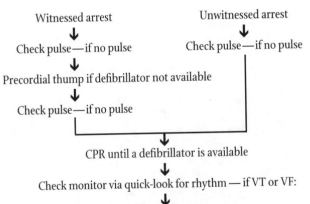

Witnessed arrest
↓
Check pulse—if no pulse
↓
Precordial thump if defibrillator not available
↓
Check pulse—if no pulse

Unwitnessed arrest
↓
Check pulse—if no pulse

↓

CPR until a defibrillator is available
↓
Check monitor via quick-look for rhythm — if VT or VF:
↓
Defibrillate with 200 joules, then 200-300 joules, then 360 joules
without pulse checks between shocks.
Confirm rhythm by monitor between defibrillations.
↓
If no pulse start CPR, intubate, establish IV access
↓
Epinephrine 1.0 mg IV Q 3-5min
or if no IV 2.0-2.5 mg in 10 ml of NS or distilled water via ET tube

(continued)

ACLS Protocols

Ventricular Fibrillation/Pulseless Ventricular Tachycardia

(continued)

↓

Defibrillate with 360 joules within 30-60sec

↓

Lidocaine 1-1.5 mg/kg IV push, may repeat Q 3-5min to max 3 mg/kg

↓

Defibrillate with 360 joules within 30-60sec

↓

Bretylium 5 mg/kg IV push,
repeat every 5min as needed, max 30-35 mg/kg

↓

Defibrillate with 360 joules within 30-60sec

↓

Magnesium sulfate 1-2 g in 10 ml IV over 1-2min

↓

Defibrillate with 360 joules within 30-60sec

↓

Procainamide 30 mg/min IV, maximum dose 17 mg/kg

↓

Defibrillate with 360 joules within 30-60sec

↓

Consider sodium bicarbonate 1 meq/kg IV

Asystole

CPR, confirm asystole in two leads, intubate, establish IV access

↓

Consider: hypoxia, hypokalemia, hyperkalemia,
hypothermia, acidosis, drug overdose

(continued)

ACLS Protocols

Asystole (continued)
↓
Consider immediate transcutaneous pacing
↓
Epinephrine 1.0 mg IV Q 3-5min,
or if no IV 2.0-2.5 mg in 10 ml NS or distilled water via ET tube
↓
Atropine 1.0 mg IV Q 3-5min, maximum total 3 mg
or if no IV 2.0-2.5 mg in 10 ml NS or distilled water via ET tube
↓
Consider sodium bicarbonate 1 meq/kg IV
↓
Consider termination of efforts

Pulseless electrical activity

Continue CPR, intubate, establish IV access
↓
Assess blood flow using Doppler
↓
Consider: hypoxia, hypokalemia, hyperkalemia, hypothermia,
acidosis, drug overdose, hypovolemia, cardiac tamponade,
massive MI, tension pneumothorax, pulmonary embolus
↓
Epinephrine 1.0 mg IV Q 3-5min,
or if no IV 2.0-2.5 mg in 10 ml NS or distilled water via ET tube
↓
Atropine 1.0 mg IV Q 3-5min,
or if no IV 2.0-2.5 mg in 10 ml NS or distilled water via ET tube
↓
Consider sodium bicarbonate 1 meq/kg IV

ACLS Protocols

Wide Complex Tachycardia of Uncertain Origin

A. _Stable patient_

Airway, **B**reathing, **C**irculation, O2, establish IV access
↓
Lidocaine 1.0-1.5 mg/kg IV, repeat 0.5-0.75 mg/kg
every 5-10min as needed, max total 3 mg/kg
↓
Adenosine 6 mg rapidly IV
↓
If tachycardia persists after 1-2min, give adenosine 12 mg rapidly IV
↓
If tachycardia persists after 1-2min, repeat adenosine 12 mg rapidly IV
↓
Procainamide 20-30 mg/min IV, max total 17 mg/kg
↓
Bretylium 5-10 mg/kg in 50 ml over 8-10min IV, max 30 mg/kg in 24h
↓
Considered synchronized countershock

B. _Unstable patient_

Airway, **B**reathing, **C**irculation, O2, establish IV access
↓
Consider treating with medications
↓
If serious signs and symptoms present, prepare for countershock
↓
Administer sedation if possible
↓
Synchronized countershock with 100J, 200J, 300J, 360J

ACLS Protocols

Sustained Ventricular Tachycardia with a Pulse

A. *Stable patient*

Airway, **B**reathing, **C**irculation, O2, establish IV access

↓

Lidocaine 1.0-1.5 mg/kg IV, repeat 0.5-0.75 mg/kg every 5-10min as needed, max total 3 mg/kg

↓

Procainamide 20-30 mg/min IV, max 17 mg/kg

↓

Bretylium 5-10 mg/kg in 50 ml over 8-10min IV, max 30 mg/kg in 24h

↓

Synchronized countershock with 100J, 200J, 300J, 360J

B. *Unstable patient*

Airway, **B**reathing, **C**irculation, O2, establish IV access

↓

Consider treating with medications

↓

If serious signs and symptoms are present, prepare for countershock

↓

Administer sedation if possible

↓

Synchronized countershock with 100J, 200J, 300J, 360J

ACLS Protocols

Polymorphic Ventricular Tachycardia

A. *Stable patient*

Treatment of choice is pacemaker

↓

Consider either:
- Magnesium sulfate 1-2 g IV over 1-2min,
  then 1-2 g over 1h as infusion **preferred**; *or*
- Isoproterenol 2-10 μg/min infusion

B. *Unstable patient, sustained arrhythmia*

Airway, **B**reathing, **C**irculation,
O2, establish IV access

↓

Consider treating with medications

↓

Administer sedation if possible

↓

Unsynchronized countershock
with 200J, 200-300J, 360J

ACLS Protocols

Symptomatic Bradycardia*

A. *Narrow QRS complex with sinus bradycardia, junctional rhythm,
   2nd degree heart block Mobitz I, or 3rd degree heart block*

Airway, **B**reathing, **C**irculation,
O₂, establish IV access

↓

Atropine 0.5-1.0 mg every 3-5min to maximum 2-3 mg

↓

Transcutaneous pacemaker

↓

Dopamine infusion 5-20 µg/kg/min; *or*
Epinephrine infusion 2-10 µg/min; *or*
Isoproterenol infusion 2-20 µg/min

B. *Wide QRS complex with 2nd degree heart block Mobitz type II
   or 3rd degree heart block*

Airway, **B**reathing, **C**irculation,
O₂, establish IV access

↓

Transcutaneous pacemaker
(prepare for transvenous pacemaker)

↓

Dopamine infusion 5-20 µg/kg/min; *or*
Epinephrine infusion 2-10 µg/min; *or*
Isoproterenol infusion 2-20 µg/min

*Symptoms = chest pain, shortness of breath, decreased conscious-
ness, shock, pulmonary vascular congestion, heart failure, acute MI.

ACLS Protocols

Atrial Fibrillation or Flutter with Rapid Ventricular Rate

A. *Stable patient*

Airway, Breathing, Circulation, O2, establish IV access

↓

Consider either:
- Diltiazem 0.25 mg/kg (20 mg) IV over 2min followed 15min later with 0.35 mg/kg (25 mg) IV over 2 min; *or*
- Atenolol 5-10 mg IV over 5min; *or*
- Esmolol 500 µg/kg over 1min, then maintenance infusion at 50 µg/kg/min over 4min (see p. 154 for dosing chart); *or*
- Metoprolol 5-10 mg slow IV push Q 5min x 3; *or*
- Propranolol 0.033 mg/kg slow IVP Q 2-3min x 3; *or*
- Verapamil 2.5-5.0 mg IV over 2min. May repeat 5-10 mg Q 15-30min, maximum total 20 mg

↓

If above fail, consider digoxin, procainamide, quinidine

B. *Unstable patient*

Airway, Breathing, Circulation, O2, establish IV access

↓

Consider treating with medications as above

↓

If serious signs and symptoms present, prepare for countershock

↓

Administer sedation if possible

↓

Atrial flutter
Synchronized countershock with 50J, 100J, 200J, 300J, 360J
Atrial fibrillation
Synchronized countershock with 100J, 200J, 300J, 360J

ACLS Protocols

Narrow QRS Complex Tachycardia (PSVT)

A. Stable patient

Airway, **B**reathing, **C**irculation, O2, establish IV access
↓
Vagal maneuvers
↓
Adenosine 6 mg rapidly IV
↓
If PSVT persists after 1-2min, give adenosine 12 mg rapidly IV
↓
If PSVT persists after 1-2min, repeat adenosine 12 mg rapidly IV
↓
If PSVT persists, verapamil 2.5-5 mg slow IV
↓
If PSVT persists after 15-30min, verapamil 5-10 mg slow IV
↓
Consider digoxin, β-blockers, diltiazem

B. Unstable patient

Airway, **B**reathing, **C**irculation, O2, establish IV access
↓
Consider treating with medications as above
↓
If serious signs and symptoms present, prepare for countershock
↓
Administer sedation if possible
↓
Synchronized countershock with 50J, 100J, 200J, 300J, 360J

Rapid Sequence Intubation

General considerations

1. *Pre-oxygenate:* if possible, allow the patient to spontaneously breathe 100% O2 for 3-5 minutes—unnecessarily assisting ventilation with a bag-mask may induce aspiration. A pulse oximeter is extremely helpful in assuring that oxygenation is adequate.

2. *Pre-treatment:* it may be desirable to omit this step under certain circumstances. For example, hypotensive patients do not require lidocaine, and waiting for the defasciculating dose to take effect may be impractical in critically ill or injured patients.

   • Vecuronium 0.01 mg/kg rapidly IV *(defasciculating dose)*; *and/or*

   • Lidocaine 1.5 mg/kg rapidly IV *(blunts rise in intracranial pressure)*

3. *Sedation:* an essential step, as it ensures the patient will not be awake while paralyzed. With the exception of sodium thiopental, sedatives should be administered at least 60 seconds before administration of paralyzing agents (thiopental is very rapidly acting and therefore a good choice when time is essential). Choice of medication is based on the clinical situation at hand.

   • Sodium thiopental 2-5 mg/kg rapidly IV *(helpful in head injured patients or patients with HTN, avoid if hypotension present)*; *or*

   • Midazolam 0.05-0.15 mg/kg rapidly IV; *or*

   • Ketamine 1.0-1.5 mg/kg rapidly IV *(helpful with status asthmaticus, avoid in head injured patients or those with cardiovascular disease)*

4. *Paralysis:* the agent of choice is succinylcholine, except for patients who may be hyperkalemic. Patients with ruptured globes should be treated with a defasciculating agent. Although there is some debate

Rapid Sequence Intubation

about the use of succinylcholine in head-injured patients, we feel it is safe in this setting. Children should be pre-treated with atropine 0.02 mg/kg to prevent bradycardia. Vecuronium has a slower onset of action than succinylcholine, as well as a considerably longer duration of action.

- Succinylcholine 1.0-1.5 mg/kg *(children up to 2 mg/kg)* rapidly IV; *or*
- Vecuronium 0.1-0.15 mg/kg rapidly IV

Detroit Receiving Hospital Rapid Sequence Intubation Protocol

Time 0-3.0 minutes   *Pre-oxygenate (continue until patient intubated):* Assemble drugs and prepare for intubation

Time 3.0-3.5 minutes   *Pre-treat if desired or needed:* Lidocaine 1.5 mg/kg rapidly IV; *and/or* Vecuronium 0.01 mg/kg rapidly IV

Time 3.5-4.0 minutes   *Administer sedation, allow 1-2 minutes for effect:* Sodium thiopental 2-5 mg/kg rapidly IV; *or* Midazolam 0.05-0.15 mg/kg rapidly IV

Time 5.0-5.5 minutes   *Administer paralytic agent and wait 1 minute:* Perform Sellick's maneuver (gentle cricoid pressure) Succinylcholine 1.0-1.5 mg/kg rapidly IV; *or* Vecuronium 0.1-0.15 mg/kg rapidly IV

Time 6.5 minutes   *Intubate*

Dobutamine Dosing

This table indicates *infusion rates in ml/hr*, assuming dobutamine 250 mg in 250 ml of D5W.
Suggested starting dose for cardiogenic shock is 0.5 µg/kg/minute.

Desired dose in µg/kg/minute

Kg	LB	1	2	3	4	5	6	7	8	9	10	12	14	15	16	18	20
1	2	0.1	0.1	0.2	0.2	0.3	0.4	0.4	0.5	0.5	0.6	0.7	0.8	0.9	1.0	1.1	1.2
2	4	0.1	0.2	0.4	0.5	0.6	0.7	0.8	1.0	1.1	1.2	1.4	1.7	1.8	1.9	2.2	2.4
5	11	0.3	0.6	0.9	1.2	1.5	1.8	2.1	2.4	2.7	3.0	3.6	4.2	4.5	4.8	5.4	6.0
10	22	0.6	1.2	1.8	2.4	3.0	3.6	4.2	4.8	5.4	6.0	7.2	8.4	9.0	10	11	12
20	44	1.2	2.4	3.6	4.8	6.0	7.2	8.4	10	11	12	14	17	18	19	22	24
30	66	1.8	3.6	5.4	7.2	9.0	11	13	14	16	18	22	25	27	29	32	36
40	88	2.4	4.8	7.2	10	12	14	17	19	22	24	29	34	36	38	43	48
50	110	3.0	6.0	9.0	12	15	18	21	24	27	30	36	42	45	48	54	60
60	132	3.6	7.2	11	14	18	22	25	29	32	36	43	50	54	58	65	72
70	154	4.2	8.4	13	17	21	25	29	34	38	42	50	59	63	67	76	84
80	176	4.8	10	14	19	24	29	34	38	43	48	58	67	72	77	86	96
90	198	5.4	11	16	22	27	32	38	43	49	54	65	76	81	86	97	108
100	220	6.0	12	18	24	30	36	42	48	54	60	72	84	90	96	108	120

Dopamine Dosing

This table indicates *infusion rates in ml/hr*, assuming dopamine 400 mg in 250 ml of D5W. If using 200 mg in 250 ml, multiply doses given below by a factor of 2. If using 800 mg in 250 ml, multiply doses given below by a factor of 0.5. Suggested starting dose for hypotension is 5 µg/kg/minute.

Desired dose in µg/kg/minute

Kg	LB	1	2	3	4	5	6	7	8	9	10	15	20	25	30	40	50
1	2	0.0	0.1	0.1	0.1	0.2	0.2	0.3	0.3	0.3	0.4	0.6	0.8	0.9	1.1	1.5	1.9
2	4	0.1	0.1	0.2	0.3	0.4	0.5	0.5	0.6	0.7	0.8	1.1	1.5	1.9	2.2	3.0	3.8
5	11	0.2	0.4	0.6	0.8	0.9	1.1	1.3	1.5	1.7	1.9	2.8	3.8	4.7	5.6	7.5	9.4
10	22	0.4	0.8	1.1	1.5	1.9	2.2	2.6	3.0	3.4	3.8	5.6	7.5	9.4	11	15	19
20	44	0.8	1.5	2.2	3.0	3.8	4.5	5.2	6.0	6.8	7.5	11	15	19	22	30	38
30	66	1.1	2.2	3.4	4.5	5.6	6.8	7.9	9.0	10	11	17	22	28	34	45	56
40	88	1.5	3.0	4.5	6.0	7.5	9.0	10	12	14	15	22	30	38	45	60	75
50	110	1.9	3.8	5.6	7.5	9.4	11	13	15	17	19	28	38	47	56	75	94
60	132	2.2	4.5	6.8	9.0	11	14	16	18	20	22	34	45	56	68	90	112
70	154	2.6	5.2	7.9	10	13	16	18	21	24	26	39	52	66	79	105	131
80	176	3.0	6.0	9.0	12	15	18	21	24	27	30	45	60	75	90	120	150
90	198	3.4	6.8	10	14	17	20	24	27	30	34	51	68	84	101	135	169
100	220	3.8	7.5	11	15	19	22	26	30	34	38	56	75	94	112	150	188

Esmolol Dosing

This table indicates *infusion rates in ml/hr*, assuming esmolol 2.5 g in 250 ml of D5W (or 5 g in 500 ml). See p. 60 for further dosing information on esmolol.

Desired dose in µg/kg/minute

Kg Pounds	13	25	38	50	63	75	88	100	113	125	138	150	163	175	188	200
40 88	3	6	9	12	15	18	21	24	27	30	33	36	39	42	45	48
45 99	4	7	10	14	17	20	24	27	31	34	37	40	44	47	51	54
50 110	4	8	11	15	19	22	26	30	34	38	41	45	49	52	56	60
55 121	4	8	13	16	21	25	29	33	37	41	46	50	54	58	62	66
60 132	5	9	14	18	23	27	32	36	41	45	50	54	59	63	68	72
65 143	5	10	15	20	25	29	34	39	44	49	54	58	64	68	73	78
70 154	5	10	16	21	26	32	37	42	47	52	58	63	68	74	79	84
75 165	6	11	17	22	28	34	40	45	51	56	62	68	73	79	85	90
80 176	6	12	18	24	30	36	42	48	54	60	66	72	78	84	90	96
85 187	7	13	19	26	32	38	45	51	58	64	70	76	83	89	96	102
90 198	7	14	21	27	34	40	48	54	61	68	75	81	88	94	102	108
95 209	7	14	22	28	36	43	50	57	64	71	79	86	93	100	107	114
100 220	8	15	23	30	38	45	53	60	68	75	83	90	98	105	113	120

Nitroprusside Dosing

This table indicates *infusion rates in ml/hr*, assuming nitroprusside 50 mg in 250 ml of D5W. Suggested starting dose for hypertensive emergency is 0.5 µg/kg/minute.

Desired dose in µg/kg/minute

Kg	LB	0.25	0.5	1	2	3	4	5	6	7	8	9	10
1	2	0.1	0.1	0.3	0.6	0.9	1.2	1.5	1.8	2.1	2.4	2.7	3.0
2	4	0.1	0.3	0.6	1.2	1.8	2.4	3.0	3.6	4.2	4.8	5.4	6.0
5	11	0.4	0.8	1.5	3.0	4.5	6.0	7.5	9.0	10	12	14	15
10	22	0.8	1.5	3.0	6.0	9.0	12	15	18	21	24	27	30
20	44	1.5	3.0	6.0	12	18	24	30	36	42	48	54	60
30	66	2.2	4.5	9.0	18	27	36	45	54	63	72	81	90
40	88	3.0	6.0	12	24	36	48	60	72	84	96	108	120
50	110	3.8	7.5	15	30	45	60	75	90	105	120	135	150
60	132	4.5	9.0	18	36	54	72	90	108	126	144	162	180
70	154	5.2	10	21	42	63	84	105	126	147	168	189	210
80	176	6.0	12	24	48	72	96	120	144	168	192	216	240
90	198	6.8	14	27	54	81	108	135	162	189	216	243	270
100	220	7.5	15	30	60	90	120	150	180	210	240	270	300

Cardiovascular Formulae

Cardiac index = cardiac output / body surface area*
Normal = 3.0 - 3.4 L / min-m^2
*See p. 165 for body surface area nomogram

Mean arterial (or pulmonary) pressure =
Diastolic pressure + ($\frac{1}{3}$ x pulse pressure)

Systemic vascular resistance =
79.92 (Mean arterial pressure – central venous pressure)
/ cardiac index
Normal = 1970 - 2390 dyne-sec / cm^5-m^2

Pulmonary vascular resistance =
79.92 (Mean pulmonary artery pressure – wedge pressure)
/ cardiac index
Normal = 255 - 285 dyne-sec / cm^5-m^2

Pressure in mmHg = pressure in cm H_2O / 1.36

Arterial blood O$_2$ content (CaO$_2$) =
(pa O$_2$ x .003) + (1.34 x Hb in gm x arterial blood Hb O$_2$ sat %)
Normal = 18 - 20 ml/dl

Venous blood O$_2$ content (CvO$_2$) =
(pv O$_2$ x .003) + (1.34 x Hb in gm x venous blood Hb O$_2$ sat %)
Normal = 13 - 16 ml/dl

Cardiovascular Formulae

Arteriovenous O2 difference (avDO2) = $(CaO_2) - (CvO_2)$
Normal = 4 - 5 ml/dl

O2 delivery index (DO2I) = CaO_2 x cardiac index x 10
Normal = 500 - 600 ml / min-m^2

O2 consumption index (VO2I) =
Arteriovenous O2 difference x cardiac index x 10
Normal = 120 - 160 ml / min-m^2

O2 extraction (O2 Ext) =
(Arteriovenous O2 difference / arterial blood O2 content) x 100
Normal = 20 - 30%

Alveolar pO2 = $[FIO_2 \times (ambient\ atmosph.\ pressure^* - 47)] - (1.2 \times paCO_2)$
* = 760 torr at sea level

Alveolar - Arterial O2 difference or "A-a gradient" or p(A-a) O2
= Alveolar pO2 – paO2
Normal < 10 torr

Shunt % = $(CcO_2 - CaO_2 / CcO_2 - CvO_2)$
CcO_2 = Hb in gm x 1.34 + (Alveolar pO2 x .003)
Normal < 10 %
Considerable disease = 20 - 29%
Life threatening > 30%

Normal Resting Hemodynamic Values

Pressure/resistance	Range
Central venous	0-6 cm H_2O
Right atrial	0-5 mmHg
Pulmonary vascular resistance	255-285 dyne-sec/cm^5-m^2
Right ventricular	
Systolic	15-30 mmHg
Diastolic	0-8 mmHg
Pulmonary arterial	
Systolic	15-30 mmHg
Diastolic	3-12 mmHg
Pulmonary wedge	3-15 mmHg
Left atrial	2-12 mmHg
Left ventricle	
Systolic	100-140 mmHg
Diastolic	3-12 mmHg
Systemic vascular resistance	1970-2390 dyne-sec/cm^5-m^2

Intravenous Fluid Components

Fluid	Volume (ml)	Na meq/l	Bicarbonate meq/l	Bicarbonate meq/ml	K meq/l	Dextrose gm/l
D5	1000	0	0	0	0	50
D10	1000	0	0	0	0	100
NS	1000	154	0	0	0	0
0.2NS/D5	1000	34	0	0	0	50
0.45NS	1000	77	0	0	0	0
3%NS	1000	513	0	0	0	0
LR*	1000	130	0*	0	4	0
D50	50	0	0	0	0	500

Na Bicarbonate

8.4%	50	1000	1000	1	0	0
7.5%	50	900	892	0.9	0	0
8.4%	10	1000	1000	1	0	0

*Also contains lactate 28 meq/l and calcium 3 mg/dl

Causes of Metabolic Acidosis

Increased anion gap*

    Diabetic ketoacidosis
    Alcoholic or starvation ketoacidosis
    Renal failure
    Intoxications
        Salicylate
        Methanol
        Ethylene glycol
        Isopropanol
        Paraldehyde
    Lactic acidosis
        Inadequate oxygen delivery
            Shock (septic or hypovolemic)
            Generalized seizures
            Carbon monoxide poisoning
            Hypoxemia
        Failure to utilize oxygen
            Phenformin
            Diabetes mellitus
            Isoniazid overdose
            Iron overdose
        Unknown causes
            Hepatic cirrhosis
            Pancreatitis
            Pregnancy, especially with toxemia
            Chronic renal failure

Normal anion gap†

    GI loss of bicarbonate
        Diarrhea
        Small bowel or pancreatic drainage or fistula
        Ureterosigmoidostomy
        Anion exchange resins
        Ingestion of $CaCl_2$ or $MgCl_2$

Causes of Metabolic Acidosis

Renal loss of bicarbonate
      Carbonic anhydrase inhibitors
      Renal tubular acidosis
      Hyperparathyroidism
      Hypoaldosteronism
Miscellaneous
      Dilutional acidosis
      Ingestion of NH_4 or HCl
      Sulfur ingestion

* (Na - Chloride - CO_2 content ≥ 16 meq / L)
† (Na - Chloride - CO_2 content < 16 meq / L)

Causes of Metabolic Alkalosis

GI disorders
      Vomiting
      Gastric drainage
      Villous adenoma of the colon
      Chloride diarrhea
Diuretic
Correction of chronic hypercapnia
Cystic fibrosis
Hyperaldosteronism
Cushing's syndrome
Bartter's syndrome
Excessive licorice intake
Severe potassium depletion
Absorbable alkali administration
Milk-alkali syndrome
Massive blood or plasma transfusion
Non-parathyroid hypercalcemia
Glucose ingestion after starvation
Large doses of carbenicillin or penicillin

Acid-Base Nomogram

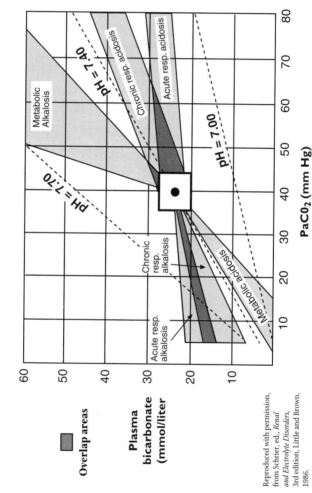

Acid-Base Nomogram

Overlap areas

Reproduced with permission, from Schrier, ed., *Renal and Electrolyte Disorders*, 3rd edition, Little and Brown, 1986.

Acid-Base Assessment Formulae

1) For **acute respiratory acidosis** or **alkalosis**:
   - *Is change in pH appropriate for acute change in paCO2?*
     $$\Delta pH \text{ (from 7.40)} = (\Delta paCO2 \text{ from 40 mm Hg}) \times .007$$

2) For **respiratory alkalosis**:
   - *Is bicarbonate concentration appropriate for change in paCO2?*

   Acute:
   Fall in HCO_3^- (from 24 mmol/l) = range of 1 to 3 × ($\Delta paCO2$ / 10)
   Bicarbonate should not fall below 18 mmol/l

   Chronic:
   Fall in HCO_3^- = range of 2 to 5 × ($\Delta paCO2$ / 10)
   Bicarbonate should not fall below 14 mmol/l

3) For **respiratory acidosis**:
   - *Is bicarbonate concentration appropriate for change in paCO2?*

   Acute:
   Rise in HCO_3^- = ($\Delta paCO2$ / 10). Appropriate range ± 3.

   Chronic:
   Rise in HCO_3^- = ($\Delta paCO2$ × 4) / 10. Appropriate range ± 4.

4) For checking the appropriateness of respiratory compensation in metabolic disorders:

   a) In **metabolic acidosis**:
      - *Is compensatory change in paCO2 appropriate for degree of acidosis as expressed by drop in bicarbonate?*
      Drop in paCO2 = range of 1.0 to 1.5 × (ΔHCO_3^- from 24 mmol/l)
      Expect paCO2 to be 26 to 36.5 mmHg

Opposite: acid-base nomogram, derived from the formulae beginning on this page. Central square = area of normality for pCO2 and bicarbonate ± 4 units. A mixed acid-base disorder should always be considered, since on the nomogram it may mimic a single acute disorder.

Acid-Base Status Assessment Formulae

b) In **metabolic alkalosis**:
  • *Is compensatory change in paCO2 appropriate for degree of alkalosis as expressed by rise in bicarbonate?*
  Δ paCO2 = range of 0.25 to 1.0 × (Δ HCO3⁻ from 24 mmol/l)

5) To calculate bicarbonate deficit in **metabolic acidosis**:
   Deficit = 0.5 × (wt in kg) × (Δ HCO3⁻ from 24 mmol/l)
   When pH < 7.1 use:
   0.8 × (wt in kg)

6) For venous blood gases:
   pvCO2 normally 6-7 mmHg more than paCO2;
   CO2 content 2.5-3.0 mmHg more than arterial;
   Bicarbonate 1 mmol/l more than arterial.

Acute Renal Failure vs. Pre-Renal Azotemia

Test	Azotemia	Renal failure
Urine osmolality	> 500	< 400 mosm/kg
Urine sodium	< 20	> 40 meq/L
Urine creatinine/plasma creatinine	> 40	< 20
Renal failure index	< 1	> 2
Fractional excretion of sodium	< 1	> 2
Urine sediment	Normal or occ granular casts	Brown granular casts, cellular debris

$$Renal\ failure\ index = \frac{U\,[Na]}{(U\,[Cr]\,/\,P\,[Cr])}$$

$$Fractional\ excretion\ of\ sodium = \frac{(U\,[Na]\,/\,P\,[Na])}{(U\,[Cr]\,/\,P\,[Cr]) \times 100}$$

U = urine   P = plasma   Na = sodium   Cr = creatinine

Body Surface Area Nomogram

Height	Surface area	Weight
in *cm*	*m²*	*lb* *kg*

To determine body surface area: find height in centimeters or inches on left-hand scale, and weight in pounds or kilograms on the right-hand scale. A straight line joining these points will cross the middle scale at the body surface area in meters squared.

Height
in — cm
80 — 200
76 — 190
72 — 180
      170
66 —
      160
60 — 150
54 — 140
      130
48 — 120
45 — 110
42 —
39 — 100
36 — 90
34 —
32 — 80
30 —
28 — 70
26 —
24 — 60
20 — 55

Surface area
m²
2.8
2.6
2.4
2.2
2.0
1.8
1.6
1.4
1.2
1.0
0.9
0.8
0.7
0.6
0.5
0.4
0.3

Weight
lb — kg
350 — 160
300 — 140
250 — 120
      100
200 — 90
      80
150 — 70
      60
120 — 50
100 — 40
90 —
80 — 35
70 — 30
60 — 25
50 — 20
40 —
35 — 15
30 —
25 — 10
20 —
15 —
      5
10 —

Pediatric Normal Peak Expiratory Flow

Mean ± 2 standard deviations

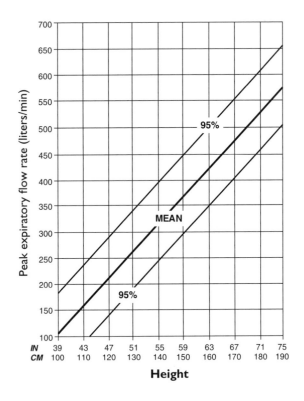

Redrawn from data obtained from 382 children age 5 to 18 years by
Godfrey et. al., *Brit J Dis Chest*, 1970; 64:15. Reproduced with
permission of Armstrong Medical Industries, Northbrook, IL.

Adult Normal Peak Expiratory Flow

By height, from age 15 to 70 years

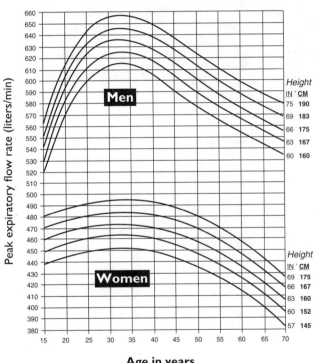

Reproduced with permission of Armstrong Medical
Industries. From Gregg and Nunn, *Br Med J*, 1973.

Hemophilia A and B Treatment

1. **Obtain an accurate history,** either from patient and relatives or from Hemophilia Treatment Center personnel, **about**:
   a. hemophilia type: 80% of patients have hemophilia A (factor VIII deficiency), 20% have hemophilia B (factor IX deficiency).
   b. *severity* of deficiency:
      1. *Severe* (<1% factor activity): frequent spontaneous bleeding.
      2. *Moderate* (2-5% factor activity): occasional spontaneous, frequent trauma-induced bleeding.
      3. *Mild* (5-20% factor activity): trauma or surgical bleeding.

2. **Replace coagulation factor *always*:**
   a. if patient has severe headache or altered mental status, *or* has sustained trauma, *or* before any invasive diagnostic procedure.
   b. unless patient has already received adequate factor dose (many patients receive self or home treatment).

3. **Selection of factor concentrates:** use specific factor VIII or factor IX clotting factor concentrate—not plasma or cryoprecipitate. All concentrates listed below are free of HIV and Hepatitis A, B, and C.
   a. **Hemophilia A** (Factor VIII deficiency—laboratory findings: prolonged PTT, decreased factor VIII level, normal factor IX.
      Factor pharmacokinetics: $T^1/_2 = 12$h.
      Dosing interval: Q 8-12h or by continuous infusion.
      Factor choices:
      Highest purity: Recombinant factor VIII (*Kogenate, Recombinate, VIII SQ*).
      High purity: *AHF-M, Hemofil-M, Monoclate-P.*
      There is *no* current indication for intermediate purity factor VIII.
      Alternatives to factor: Desmopressin (*DDAVP, Stimate*): 0.3 ug/kg in 50 ml 0.9% saline over 30min for pts with mild-moderate disease (use with caution in pts >50 y.o. or with cardiac histories).
   b. **Hemophilia A with Inhibitor** (consult hematology)—laboratory findings: prolonged PTT, decreased factor VIII activity, positive factor VIII inhibitor study.
      Factor pharmacokinetics: uncertain—factor concentrates are intended to bypass or saturate antibody to factor VIII.

Hemophilia A and B Treatment

Dosing interval: Q 8-12h.
Factor choices: Recombinant VIIa; activated factor IX complex
    (*FEIBA, Autoplex*); non-activated IX (*Konyne 80*); high-dose
    continuous infusion factor VIII.

c. **Hemophilia B** (Factor IX deficiency)—laboratory findings:
    prolonged PTT, decreased factor IX activity. (Hemophilia B
    patients may also exhibit inhibitors, manifested by abnormal
    mixing studies and positive factor IX inhibitor assay.)
    Factor pharmacokinetics: T$^1/_2$ = 18-24h.
    Dosing interval: Q 12-24h.
    Factor choices: *Alphanine, Konyne 80, Mononine.*

4. **Dosing of factor—appropriate for all concentrates:**
    a. *Life-threatening bleeds* (intracranial or retroperitoneal hemorrhage,
       major trauma or surgery): 40-50 U/kg IV bolus, then 5- 10 U/kg/h
       by continous infusion.
    b. *"Routine" bleeds* (hemarthroses, hematuria, minor soft tissue):
       20-25 U/kg bolus, repeat Q 12-18h as necessary.

5. **Do not:** refrain from indicated invasive diagnostic procedures—
    administer factor concentrate, then proceed as indicated by patient's
    clinical condition. **Avoid:** unnecessary invasive procedures, IM
    injections, aspirin and other NSAIDs for pain relief. **Use:** adequate
    measures for pain control.

6. **A history of clotting factor "inhibitor"** (antibody) requires special
    measures (special concentrates, urgent hematology consultation).

7. Women *can* have hemophilia. Patients usually know about their
    disease and its treatment—it pays to listen to them. The hemophilias
    are X-linked recessive disorders, but since 40% of cases occur by
    spontaneous mutation, a family history of hemophilia may be absent.

8. If available, obtain hematology consultation while patient is in ED; at DC
    refer patient to a Hemophilia Treatment Center. Obtain listings from
    National Hemophilia Foundation, phone (212) 219-8180, *M-F 9 a.m.-
    5 p.m. EST* or Hemophilia Foundation of Michigan, (313) 761-2535.

Von Willebrand's Disease Treatment

Etiology:

Deficiency or dysfunction of von Willebrand factor, a large plasma transport protein for factor VIII that also promotes platelet adhesion and tissue healing. Autosomal dominant inheritance.

Symptoms:

Excessive bruising, epistaxis, gingival or GI bleeding, hematuria, hypermenorrhea.

Laboratory findings:

Prolonged bleeding time, decreased factor VIIIc level, decreased vWF activity and antigen.

Treatment:

1. Desmopressin (*DDAVP, Stimate*): Concentrated nasal spray or IV preparation (0.3 ug/kg in 50 cc 0.9% NaCl over 30min; use with caution in patients >50 y.o. or with previous history of MI); *or*

2. *Humate P:* 25-30 U/kg IV Q 24h; *or*

3. Cryoprecipitate ("pedigree" only): 1 unit (bag) per 5 kg of patient weight Q 12-24h as indicated (may transmit virus undetected by clinical testing); *or*

4. Von Willebrand factor concentrate: not yet available in US, but is in European clinical trials (see literature for dose).

Remember: Von Willebrand's appears equally frequently in men and women but women have more frequent symptoms because of menstrual bleeding; inhibitors occur but are relatively infrequent.

Catheter Clearance Protocol

1. Ascertain that catheter occlusion is not due to venous thrombosis or infection.

2. Use appropriate aseptic and anti-embolic precautions for central venous catheters.

3. Use urokinase to avoid patient sensitization to streptokinase, in case systemic administration of thrombolytic becomes necessary.

4. Draw into smallest syringe possible 5,000 to 15,000 units (1-3 ml) of urokinase for each catheter lumen, according to catheter type and volume.

5. Have patient, in supine position, exhale and hold breath while catheter is open. Uncap catheter using aseptic technique, attach empty syringe, and aspirate gently.

6. If no blood return achieved, replace empty syringe with urokinase-filled one, aspirate gently, then slowly inject urokinase. Recap catheter, allow to remain 60-120 minutes, then uncap and gently re-aspirate. If blood return is achieved, draw 5-10 cc of blood, flush catheter with 100 cc of saline, then refill with heparinized saline (1000 U heparin/cc), then recap.

7. If no blood return is achieved after 120 mins, refill catheter with urokinase reconstituted to achieve 40,000-70,000 U/lumen, allow to remain for 120 min., then reaspirate and flush, as above, if blood return is achieved. If no return is achieved, leave solution in place for additional 12 hours, attempt to reaspirate and, if successful, flush.

8. Failure to clear catheter after 12 hours suggests either organized thrombus unlikely to be dissolved with additional thrombolytic agent, or anatomic abnormality. Angiography may be helpful in determining catheter viability.

9. This protocol is safe if used as outlined, even in patients with coagulopathy or thrombocytopenia.

Isolation Strategies and Contagious Periods for Infectious Diseases

SR = single room   M = mask   Go = gown   Gl = gloves   Routine = universal precautions

DISEASE	PRECAUTIONS	CONTAGIOUS PERIOD
AIDS	Routine	Blood and body fluids should be considered infective with parenteral exposure
Campylobacter	* §	Until organisms can no longer be isolated from stool
Cholera	* §	Unknown
Clostridial myonecrosis	§	Until lesions are no longer draining
Diphtheria	SR, M, Go, Gl	Until 2 cultures 24h apart from both nose/throat are negative
H. influenzae	SR, M	Until 24h after initiation of effective antibiotic therapy
H. simplex		
Neonatal	SR, M§	Duration of illness
Mucocutaneous	SR, M§	For severe cases only—duration of illness
CNS	Routine	Special precautions unnecessary
Hepatitis A	* §	From 2wks prior to symptoms; minimal 1wk after onset jaundice
Hepatitis B & C	Routine	HBsAg+ state indicates infectivity for Hepatitis B
Influenza	SR, M§	Duration of illness
Measles	SR, M	From 7d after exposure to 4d after onset of rash
Meningococcus	SR, M	Until 24h after initiation of effective antibiotic therapy
Mumps	SR, M	From 7d prior to parotid swelling to 9d after first symptoms
Pertussis	SR, M	From first sx to 3wks later or 5d after start of erythromycin

Plague	SR, M, Go, Gl	Until 72h after initiation of effective antibiotic therapy
Rabies	SR, M, Go, Gl	Duration of illness
Rubella	SR, M#	From 7d after exposure to 7d after onset of rash
Congenital	SR, M#	Until 1 year of age unless nasopharyngeal and urine cultures are negative after 3 months of age
Salmonellosis	* §	Until 3 stools after cessation of antibiotics are negative
Shigellosis	* §	Until 3 stools after cessation of antibiotics are negative
Staph ylococcus		
Pneumonia	SR, M§	Until 48h after start of effective antibiotic therapy
Skin	SR, M§	Until open wounds have resolved
Strep skin (Group A)	.. §	Until 24h after initiation of effective antibiotic therapy
Tuberculosis	SR, M	From onset of sx until drug treatment reduces organisms found in sputum and cough is decreased
Varicella		
Chicken pox	SR, M, Go, Gl	From 24h prior to rash until all lesions are crusted
Local zoster	§†	Until rash has resolved
Dissem. zoster	SR, M, Go, Gl	Until rash has resolved
Yersiniosis	* §	Unknown

* SR for patients with fecal incontinence or poor hygiene only
§ Go, Gl only if contact with infective material likely
† Add SR, M if immunocompromised
# Add Go, Gl if immunocompromised

Synovial Fluid in Acute Arthritis

Diagnosis	Appearance	WBC / mm³	PMN %	Sugar*
Normal	Straw-colored, clear	< 200	< 25	~ 100
Degenerative joint disease	Slightly turbid	< 2,000	< 25	~ 100
Traumatic arthritis	Straw-colored, bloody, or xanthochromic	~ 2,000	< 25	~ 100
Rheumatoid arthritis	Turbid	5,000-50,000	> 65	~ 75
Other types of inflammatory arthritis	Turbid	5,000-50,000	> 50	~ 75
Acute gout or pseudogout	Turbid	5,000-50,000	> 75	~ 90
Septic arthritis	Very turbid or purulent	10,000-100,000	> 80	< 50
Tuberculous arthritis	Turbid	~ 25,000	Variable	< 50

* % of blood level

With permission, from *Principles of Internal Medicine*, 10th ed, McGraw-Hill, 1976.

7
Pediatric Reference

Immunization Schedule

Oral polio vaccine	Diphtheria and tetanus toxoid/pertussis vaccine	Haemophilus influenzae B Type B conjugate vaccine	Hepatitis B virus vaccine	Live measles, mumps, rubella viruses vaccine	Adult tetanus booster	
			x			*Birth*
			x			*1-2 mo.*
x	x	x				*2 mo.*
x	x	x				*4 mo.*
	x	x¹				*6 mo.*
x			x			*6-18 mo.*
		x		x		*12-15 mo.*
	x					*15-18 mo.*
x	x					*4-6 yr*
				x		*11-12 yr*
					x	*Q 10 yr*

¹ 6 mo. dose not indicated if product in doses 1-2 was *Pedvax HIB* (PRP-OMP).

Recommended ages are not absolute—for ex., 2 mo. may be 6-10 weeks. However, do not give MMR to children < 1 y.o. If measles vacc. is indicated at < 1 y.o., give monovalent measles vaccine, then MMR at 12-15 mo.

APGAR Scoring

Criterion	0	1	2
Heart rate	Absent	< 100	> 100
Respiratory	Absent	Slow or irregular	Good crying
Muscle tone	Limp	Some flexion of extremities	Active motion
Reflex irritability (catheter in nares)	No response	Grimace	Cough or sneeze
Color	Blue, pale	Extremities blue, body pink	Completely pink

Take at 1 and 5min after birth. 8-10: normal infant; 4-7: mild-moderate impairment; 0-3: severely depressed.

Tube and Laryngoscope Sizes

Age	ET tube* (in mm)	Blade	Levine	Foley (French)	Chest tube Air (French)	Chest tube Fluid (French)
Neonatal	3.0	0	8	5-6	10-12	12
6 months	3.5-4.0	1	10	8-10	12	16-20
1 year	4.0-4.5	1	10	8-10	12-16	16-20
2 years	4.5-5.0	2	12	8-10	12-16	16-20
4 years	5.0-5.5	2	14	8-10	16-20	20-25
6 years	5.5-6.0	2	14	8-10	16-20	20-25
8 years	6.0-6.5	2-3	14	10-12	16-20	20-25
10 years	6.5-7.0	3	16	10-12	16-20	20-25
12 years	7.0-7.5	3	16	10-12	24-28	28-32
14 years	7.5-8.0	3	18	12-16	24-28	28-32

*Uncuffed tube unless > 10 years old or tube size > 6.0 mm

See also p. 178

Hematologic Indices by Age

Age	Hb (gm)*	Hct*	MCV*	WBC /mm³*
Term	13.5-20	42-60	98-118	9-30
2 weeks	13.4-19.8	41-65	88-122	5-20
1 month	10.7-17.1	33-55	91-111	5-19.5
2 months	9.4-13	28-42	84-106	5-19.5
6 months	11.1-14.1	31-41	68-84	6-17.5
6 mo.-2 yrs	10.5-13.5	33-39	70-86	6-17
2-6 yrs	11.5-13.5	34-41	75-87	5-15.5
6-12 yrs	11.5-15.5	35-45	77-95	4.5-13.5
12-18 yrs				
Male	13-16	36-50	78-98	4.5-13.5
Female	12-16	37-45	78-102	4.5-13.5

*Ranges represent ±2 SD about mean

See also p. 179

Vital Signs by Age

Age	Wt (kg)	Heart Rate	Resp Rate	Blood Pressure Syst.	Diast.
Newborn	1-2	135	< 40	40-60	20-36
Newborn	2-3	125	< 40	50-70	29-45
1 month	4	120	24-35	64-96	30-62
6 months	7	130	24-35	60-118	50-70
1 year	10	125	20-30	66-126	41-91
2-3 years	12-14	115	20-30	74-124	39-89
4-5 years	16-18	100	20-30	79-119	45-85
6-8 years	20-26	100	12-25		
10-12 years	32-42	75	12-25	See page	
> 14 years	> 50	70	12-18	179	

Hemoglobin and MCV by Age

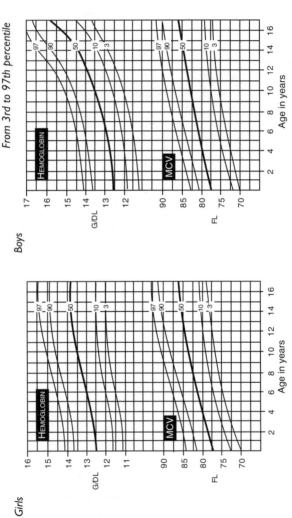

Reproduced with permission of the C.V. Mosby Co., from Dallman PR, Siimes MA: Percentile Curves for Hemoglobin and Red Cell Volume in Infancy and Childhood. *J Pediatrics* 1979; 94:26.

Normal Blood Pressure by Age

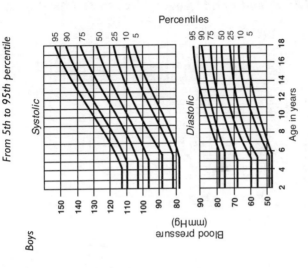

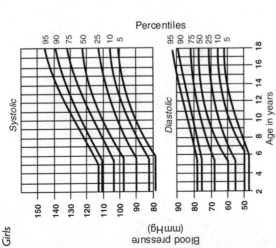

Reproduced by permission of *Pediatrics* 1977; 59 (suppl):802.

Girls' Weight and Length Birth to 36 Months

From 5th to 95th percentile

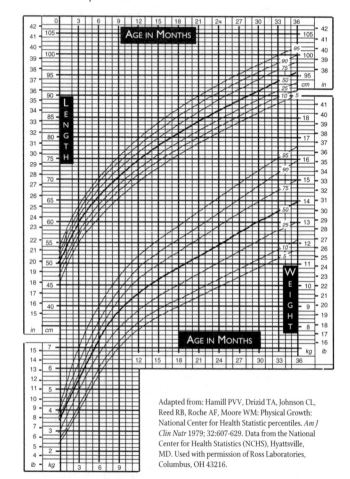

Adapted from: Hamill PVV, Drizid TA, Johnson CL, Reed RB, Roche AF, Moore WM: Physical Growth: National Center for Health Statistic percentiles. *Am J Clin Nutr* 1979; 32:607-629. Data from the National Center for Health Statistics (NCHS), Hyattsville, MD. Used with permission of Ross Laboratories, Columbus, OH 43216.

Boys' Weight and Length Birth to 36 Months

From 5th to 95th percentile

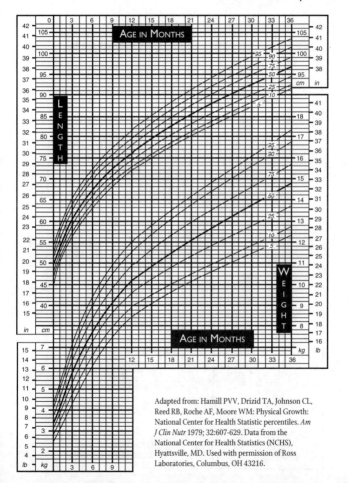

Adapted from: Hamill PVV, Drizid TA, Johnson CL, Reed RB, Roche AF, Moore WM: Physical Growth: National Center for Health Statistic percentiles. *Am J Clin Nutr* 1979; 32:607-629. Data from the National Center for Health Statistics (NCHS), Hyattsville, MD. Used with permission of Ross Laboratories, Columbus, OH 43216.

Girls' Weight and Height 2 to 18 Years

From 5th to 95th percentile

Adapted from: Hamill PVV, Drizid TA,
Johnson CL, Reed RB, Roche AF, Moore WM:
Physical Growth: National Center for Health
Statistic percentiles. *Am J Clin Nutr* 1979;
32:607-629. Data from the National Center for
Health Statistics (NCHS), Hyattsville, MD.
Used with permission of Ross Laboratories,
Columbus, OH 43216.

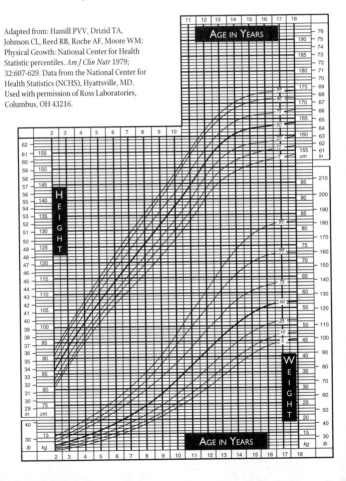

Boys' Weight and Height 2 to 18 Years

From 5th to 95th percentile

Adapted from: Hamill PVV, Drizid TA,
Johnson CL, Reed RB, Roche AF, Moore WM:
Physical Growth: National Center for Health
Statistic percentiles. *Am J Clin Nutr* 1979;
32:607-629. Data from the National Center for
Health Statistics (NCHS), Hyattsville, MD.
Used with permission of Ross Laboratories,
Columbus, OH 43216.

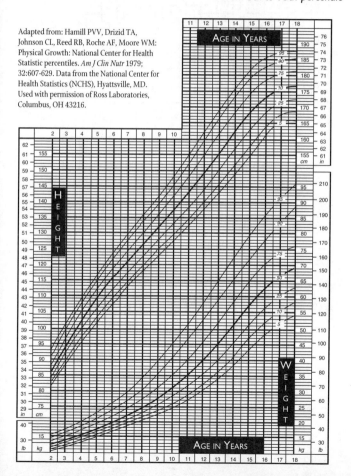

Girls' Head Circumference

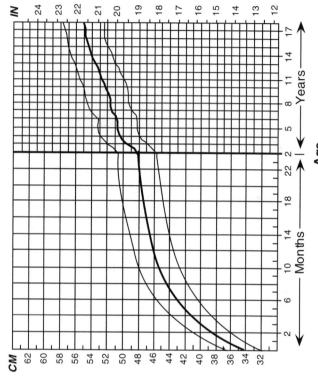

Mean ± 2 SD (2nd to 98th percentile) of head circumference for girls from birth to 18 years.

Boys'
Head
Circumference

Mean ± 2 SD (2nd to 98th percentile) of head circumference for boys from birth to 18 years.

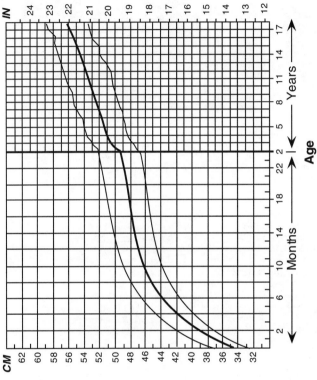

Reproduced by permission of
Pediatrics 1968; 41:106.

Major references in **bold type**
Proprietary drug names in *italic type*

Index

A

A-a gradient **157**
Accupril. See Quinapril
Acebutolol 1, **36**, 106
Acetaminophen 1, **36**
  overdose 37, **128**
    nomogram **125**
Acetaminophen/codeine 1, **36**, 106
Acetazolamide 1, 13, **36**
Acetohexamide 1, **36**
Acetylcysteine 1, **37**, 125, 128
Acid-base
  formulae **163**
  nomogram **162**
Acidosis
  metabolic **160-164**
  respiratory **162-163**
AIDS, isolation for 172
Activase. See Alteplase
Acyclovir 1, 15, **34**, **37**, 106
Adalat. See Nifedipine
Adapin. See Doxepin
Addison's disease **6**
Adenocard. See Adenosine
Adenosine 1, **37**, 144, 149
Adrenal insufficiency **6**
ACLS protocols
  Asystole **142**, **143**
  Atrial fibrillation **148**
  Atrial flutter **148**
  Bradycardia **147**
  Electromechanical dissociation **143**
  Heart block **147**
  Pulseless electrical activity **143**
  Supraventricular tachycardia **149**
  Ventricular fibrillation **141**, **142**
  Ventricular tachycardia **141**, **142**,
    144, **145**, **146**
  Wide complex tachycardia **144**
Advil. See Ibuprofen

Aerobid. See Flunisolide
Ak-Zol. See Acetazolamide
Albumin 1, **37**
Albuterol 1, **37**, 106
Alcohols
  ethanol
    dosing of **130**
    overdose 123
    withdrawal, treatment of **6**
  ethylene glycol 123, 127, **130**
  isopropanol 123, 127, 160
  methanol 123, 127, **130**, 160
Aldactazide. See Hydrochlorothiazide/
    spironolactone
Aldactone. See Spironolactone
Aldomet. See Methyldopa
Alkalosis
  metabolic **161**, **162**, **164**
  respiratory **162-163**
Allopurinol 1, **37**
Alprazolam 1, **38**
Altace. See Ramipril
Alteplase 1, **38**
Alternajel. See Aluminum hydroxide
Alu-Cap. See Aluminum hydroxide
Alu-Tab. See Aluminum hydroxide
Aluminum hydroxide 1, **38**
Alupent. See Metaproterenol
Alveolar pO2 **157**
Amantidine 1, **38**
Ambien. See Zolpidem tartrate
Amcil. See Ampicillin
Amikacin 1, 6, 7, 9, 10, 23, 25, 26, 28,
    29, 33, **38**
Amikin. See Amikacin
Amiloride 1, **39**, 106
Aminophylline 1, 6, **39**
  overdose 127
Amiodarone 1, **39**
Amitriptyline 1, **39**
Amlodipine 1, **39**, 106
Amox. See Amoxicillin
Amoxapine 1, **39**

Amoxicillin   1, 9, 11, 16, 32, **39**, 106
Amoxicillin/clavulanate   1, 7, 8, 12, 17, 25, 28, 29, 32, **40**, 106
Amphetamine overdose   126
Amphotericin   19
Ampicillin   1, 7, 10, 11, 18, 23, 25, 28, 29, 32, **40**, 106
Ampicillin/sulbactam   1, 7, 12, 23, 25, 26, 28, 32, **40**
Amyl nitrite perles   **129**
Anaphylaxis   **6**
Ancef. See Cefazolin
Ancobon. See Flucytosine
Ancylostoma duodenale   **35**
Anectine. See Succinylcholine
Anemia, iron deficiency   61, 62
Anion gap   160
Anistreplase   1, **40**
Ansaid. See Flurbiprofen
Ansamycin. See Rifabutin
Anspor. See Cephradine
Antabuse. See Disulfiram
Anticholinergic
    toxidrome   **126**
Antidotes to poisonings   **128-130**
Antiminth. See Pyrantel pamoate
Antipyrine/benzocaine   1, **40**
Antivert. See Meclizine
Aortic dissection   **6**
APGAR scoring   **176**
Apresoline. See Hydralazine
Arteriovenous oxygen difference   **157**
Arthritis
    degenerative   174
    gouty   **14**, 174
    Lyme   **17**
    pseudogout   174
    rheumatoid   174
    septic   **6**, 174
    traumatic   174
    tuberculous   174
Ascaris lumbricoides   **35**
Asendin. See Amoxapine

Aspirin   1, 21, **41**
    overdose
        nomogram   **124**
Astemizole   1, **41**, 106
Asthma   **166, 167**
Asystole   **142, 143**
Atabrine. See Quinacrine
Atenolol   1, **41**, 106, 148
Ativan. See Lorazepam
Atlanto-dental interval   118
Atovaquone   1, 24, **41**
Atracurium   1, **41**
Atrial fibrillation   **148**
Atrial flutter   **148**
Atrioventricular block. *See* Heart block
Atropine   1, 20, **41**, 88, 131, 143, 147
    for carbamate overdose   129
    for organophosphate/carbamate
        poisoning   126
Atrovent. See Ipratropium bromide
Augmentin. See Amoxicillin/clavulanate
Auralgan. See Antipyrine/benzocaine
Axid. See Nizatidine
Azactam. See Aztreonam
Azithromycin   1, 8, 9, 17, 25, 26, **42**, 106
Azmacort. See Triamcinolone
Azotemia   **164**
AZT. See Zidovudine
Aztreonam   1, 7, **42**
Azulfidine. See Sulfasalazine

B

Bacitracin   105
Baclofen   1, **42**
Bacterial vaginosis   **33**
Bactocil. See Oxacillin
Bactrim. See Trimethoprim/
    sulfamethoxazole
Bactroban. See Mupirocin
Barbita. See Phenobarbital
Bat bite   **7**
Beclomethasone   1, **42**, 106
Beclovent. See Beclomethasone

Beconase. See Beclomethasone
Belladonna   88
Bellergal-S. See Phenobarbital/ergotamine
Benadryl. See Diphenhydramine
Benazepril   1, **42**, 106
Benemid. See Probenecid
Bentyl. See Dicyclomine
Benzodiazepine overdose   63, **128**
Benztropine mesylate   1, **42**, 106, 131
Bepridil   1, **42**, 106
Beta-blocker overdose   **128**
Betapace. See Sotalol
Betaxolol   1, **43**, 106
Bethanechol   1, **43**
Biaxin. See Clarithromycin
Bicarbonate   1, **43**, 142, 143, 159
    deficit   **164**
    for quinidine overdose   **131**
    for tricyclic overdose   **129**
Biltricide. See Praziquantel
Bisacodyl   1, **43**, 106
Bisoprolol   1, **43**, 106
Bites, treatment of   **7**
Bitolterol   1, **43**, 106
Blocadren. See Timolol
Blood pressure, by age   **177**
Body surface area nomogram   **165**
Botulism   128
Bowel perforation   **23**
Bradycardia   **147**
Breast infection   **17**
Breathine. See Terbutaline
Bretylium   1, **43**, 142, 144, 145
Bretylol. See Bretylium
Brevibloc. See Esmolol
Bricanyl. See Terbutaline
Bronkosol. See Isoetharine
Bumetanide   1, **43**, 106
Bumex. See Bumetanide
Burns   **138**
BuSpar. See Buspirone
Buspirone   1, **44**
Butazolidin. See Phenylbutazone
Butoconazole   1, 33, **44**

Butorphanol   1, **44**

C

Cafergot. See Ergotamine/caffeine
Calan. See Verapamil
Calcitriol   1, **44**
Calcium channel blocker
    overdose   **128**
Calcium chloride   1, **44**, 128
Calcium gluconate   1, **44**
Campylobacter
    infection   12
    isolation for   172
Candida
    infection   8
    vaginitis   **33**
Capoten. See Captopril
Capsaicin   1, **44**, 106
Captopril   1, **44**, 106
Carafate. See Sucralfate
Carbamate poisoning   **126**, 129
Carbamazepine   2, **45**, 106
Carbaryl   126
Carbenicillin   2, 26, 28, 29, 32, 33, **45**
Carbon monoxide   160
Cardene. See Nicardipine
Cardiac index   **156**
Cardiac output   156
Cardiopulmonary resuscitation   141,
    142, 143
Cardioquin. See Quinidine
Cardiovascular formulae   **156**, **157**
Cardizem. See Diltiazem
Cardura. See Doxazosin
Carisoprodol   2, **45**
Carteolol   2, **45**, 106
Cartrol. See Carteolol
Cat bite   **7**
Catapres. See Clonidine
Catheter clearance protocol   **171**
Ceclor. See Cefaclor
Cefaclor   2, **45**, 106
Cefadroxil   2, **45**, 107
Cefadyl. See Cephapirin

Cefamandole 2, **46**
Cefazolin 2, **46**
Cefixime 2, **46**, 107
Cefizox. See Ceftizoxime
Cefmetazole 2, **46**
Cefobid. See Cefoperazone
Cefonicid 2, **46**
Cefoperazone 2, 22, 26, 29, 33, **46**
Cefotan. See Cefotetan
Cefotaxime 2, 6, 7, 12, 17, 18, 19, 25, 26, 28, 29, **46**
Cefotetan 2, 13, 22, **47**
Cefoxitin 2, 7, 9, 22, 23, 26, 28, **47**
Cefpodoxime 2, 32, **47**, 107
Cefprozil 2, **47**, 107
Ceftazidime 2, 19, 22, 26, 29, 33, **47**
Ceftin. See Cefuroxime
Ceftizoxime 2, 13, 14, **47**
Ceftriaxone 2, 7, 12, 13, 14, 17, 18, 19, 22, 25, 26, 28, 29, **47**
Cefuroxime 2, 16, 17, 21, 24, 26, 28, 29, **48**, 107
Cefzil. See Cefprozil
Celontin. See Methsuximide
Central venous pressure 158
Cephalexin 2, 32, **48**, 107
Cephalothin 2, **48**
Cephapirin 2, **48**
Cephradine 2, **48**, 107
Cephulac. See Lactulose
Cerebral edema **8**
Cerumen impaction 40
Cervical spine
    fractures, stable vs. unstable **119**
    x-ray parameters **118**
Cervicitis
    gonococcal **13**
Cesol. See Praziquantel
Charcoal, activated **121**
Chest tube sizes
    pediatric **176**
Chicken pox
    treatment **34**
    isolation for 173

Chlamydia **8**
Chlor-Trimeton. See Chlorpheniramine
Chloral hydrate 2, **48**
Chloramphenicol 2, 12, 18, 25, **49**
Chlordiazepoxide 2, **49**
Chlordiazepoxide/clidinium 2, **49**
Chloromycetin. See Chloramphenicol
Chlorothiazide 2, **49**
Chlorpheniramine 2, **49**
Chlorpromazine 2, **50**
Chlorpropamide 2, **50**, 107
Chlorthalidone 2, **50**, 107
Chlorzoxazone 2, **50**
Cholera
    isolation for 172
    treatment **13**
Cholestyramine 2, **50**
Cholinergic
    toxidrome **126**
Chromium, skin exposure to 122
Cibalith. See Lithium
Cimetidine 2, **51**, 107
Cinobac. See Cinoxacin
Cinoxacin 2, 32, **51**, 107
Cipro. See Ciprofloxacin
Ciprofloxacin 2, 7, 9, 12, 13, 14, 19, 21, 22, 27, 32, 33, **51**, 107
    eyedrops **105**
Cisapride 2, **51**, 107
Claforan. See Cefotaxime
Clarithromycin 2, 9, 17, 25, 26, 29, **51**, 107
Cleocin. See Clindamycin
Clindamycin 2, 9, 11, 17, 21, 22, 24, 25, 26, 28, 33, **51**, 107
Clinoril. See Sulindac
Clonazepam 2, **51**
Clonidine 2, **51**, 107
Clorazepate 2, **52**
Clostridial myonecrosis 172
Clostridium difficile **12**
Clotrimazole 2, 8, 9, 30, 33, **52**, 107
Cloxacillin 2, 7, 17, **52**, 107
Cloxapen. See Cloxacillin

Cocaine overdose   126
Codeine   2, **52**, 107
Codoxy. See Oxycodone/aspirin
Cogentin. See Benztropine mesylate
Cognex. See Tacrine
Colace. See Docusate sodium
Colchicine   2, **14**, **52**
Colestid. See Colestipol
Colestipol   2, **52**
Colistin   12
Coma Scale, Glasgow
    adult   **135**
    pediatric   **137**
Compazine. See Prochloperazine
Contagious periods for infectious
    diseases   **172**
Cordarone. See Amiodarone
Corgard. See Nadolol
Cortisporin. See Neomycin/polymixin B/
    hydrocortisone
Coumadin. See Warfarin
Coumarin overdose   129
Crabs   **16**
Cromolyn sodium   2, **52**
Crotamiton   2, **28**, **53**
Cryptococcal meningitis   **18**
Cyanide poisoning   **129**
Cyclic antidepressant overdose   **129**
Cyclobenzaprine   2, **53**, 107
Cyclopentolate   105
Cyproheptadine   2, **53**
Cystitis   **32**
Cytomel. See Liothyronine
Cytotec. See Misoprostol
Cytovene. See Ganciclovir

D

Dapsone   2, **24**, 25, **53**
Daranide. See Dichlorphenamide
Daraprim. See Pyrimethamine
Darvocet. See Propoxyphene/acetami-
    nophen
Darvon. See Propoxyphene
Daypro. See Oxaprozin

DDI. See Didanosine
Decadron. See Dexamethasone
Deep venous thrombosis   **34**
Deferoxamine   2, **53**, **130**
Demerol. See Meperidine
Dental anatomy   **111**
Depakene. See Valproic acid
Deponit. See Nitroglycerin
Dermatomes, sensory   **116-117**
Dermatophytosis. *See* Tinea
Desferol. See Deferoxamine
Dexamethasone   2, 8, **53**
Dextromethorphan   2
Dextrose   2, **53**
Di-Azo. See Phenazopyridine
DiaBeta. See Glyburide
Diabetes mellitus
    ketoacidosis   **9**
Diabinese. See Chlorpropamide
Diamox. See Acetazolamide
Diarrhea, infectious   **13**
Diazepam   2, 6, 9, **53**
Dichlorphenamide   2, **54**
Diclofenac   2, **54**
Dicloxacillin   2, 7, 17, **54**, 107
Dicyclomine   2, **54**
Didanosine   2, **54**
Diflucan. See Fluconazole
Diflunisal   2, **54**, 107
Digibind. See Digoxin immune FAB
Digitalis overdose   **130**
Digoxin   2, **55**
Digoxin immune FAB   2, **55**, **130**
Dihydroergotamine   2, **14**, **55**
Dilacor XR. See Diltiazem
Dilantin. See Phenytoin
Dilatrate. See Isosorbide dinitrate
Diltiazem   2, **55**, 107, 148
Dimenhydrinate   2, **56**
Dimetabs. See Dimenhydrinate
Diphenhydramine   2, 6, 9, **56**, 108, 131
Diphenoxylate/atropine   2, **56**, 108
Diphtheria
    isolation for   172

prophylaxis **23**
treatment **23**
vaccine **175**
Diphyllobothrium lathium **35**
Dipyridamole 2, **56**
Disalcid. See Salsalate
Disopyramide 2, **56**
Dissection, aortic **6**
Disulfiram 2, **56**
Ditropan. See Oxybutynin
Diulo. See Metolazone
Diuril. See Chlorothiazide
Diverticulitis **9**
Dobutamine 2, **57**
dosing chart **152**
Dobutrex. See Dobutamine
Docusate 2, **57**
Dog bite **7**
Dolobid. See Diflunisal
Dolophine. See Methadone
Done nomogram **124**
Donnatal. See Phenobarbital/hyos-
cyamine
Dopamine 2, **57**, 147
dosing chart **153**
Dopastat. See Dopamine
Doxacurium 2, **57**
Doxazosin 2, **57**, 108
Doxepin 2, **57**
Doxychel. See Doxycycline
Doxycycline 2, 7, 17, 22, 27, 30, 31, **57**, 108
Dramamine. See Dimenhydrinate
Dulcolax. See Bisacodyl
Duodenal ulcer
treatment of H. pylori **9**
Duricef. See Cefadroxil
Duvoid. See Bethanecol
Dyazide. See Hydrochlorothiazide/
triamterene
Dymelor. See Acetohexamide
DynaCirc. See Isradipine
Dynapen. See Dicloxacillin
Dyrenium. See Triamterene

Dysfunctional uterine bleeding **9**
Dystonic reaction **9**, 42

E

E-mycin. See Erythromycin
E.E.S. See Erythromycin
Eclampsia **9**
Edrophonium **20**
Eflornithine 2, **58**
Elavil. See Amitriptyline
Electromechanical dissociation **143**
Elimite. See Permethrin
Eminase. See Anistreplase
Enalapril 2, **58**, 108
Encephalitis, herpes simplex **15**
Endocarditis
gonococcal **14**
prophylaxis **10**
treatment **10**
Endotracheal tube sizes
pediatric **176**
Enduron. See Methyclothiazide
Engerix-B. See Hepatitis B vaccine
Enoxacin 2, 32, **58**
Enterobius vermicularis **35**
Epididymitis **12**
Epiglottitis **12**
Epinephrine 2, 6, **58**, 141, 143, 147
eyedrops **105**
Epinephrine, racemic 2, **58**
Ergomar. See Ergotamine
Ergostat. See Ergotamine
Ergotamine 2, **58**, 88
Ergotamine/caffeine 2, **59**
Eryc. See Erythromycin
Eryped. See Erythromycin
Erythrocin. See Erythromycin
Erythromycin 2, 3, 8, 9, 11, 16, 23, 25, 26, **59-60**, 108
Erythromycin/sulfisoxazole 3, 29, **60**, 108
Esidrix. See Hydrochlorazide
Eskalith. See Lithium

Esmolol   3, **60**, 148
    dosing chart   **154**
Esophagitis, candida   8
Ethambutol   3, **60**
Ethanol
    dosing of   130
    overdose   123
    withdrawal   **6**
Ethionamide   3, **60**
Ethmozine. See Moricizine
Ethosuximide   3, **60**
Ethril. See Erythromycin
Ethril 500. See Erythromycin
Ethylene glycol   123, 127, **130**, 160
Etodolac   3, **61**
Eye medications   **105**

F

Famciclovir   34, **61**, 108
Famotidine   3, **61**, 108
Famvir. See Famciclovir
Fansidar. See Sulfadoxine/pyrimethamine
Feldene. See Piroxicam
Felodipine   3, **61**
Femiron. See Ferrous fumarate
Femstat. See Butoconazole
Fenoprofen   3, **61**
Fentanyl   3, **61**
Feosol. See Ferrous sulfate
Feostat. See Ferrous fumarate
Fer-IN-Sol. See Ferrous sulfate
Fer-Iron. See Ferrous sulfate
Fergon. See Ferrous gluconate
Fero-Gradumet. See Ferrous sulfate
Ferospace. See Ferrous sulfate
Ferra-TD. See Ferrous sulfate
Ferralet. See Ferrous gluconate
Ferralyn. See Ferrous sulfate
Ferrous fumarate   3, **61**
Ferrous gluconate   3, **62**
Ferrous sulfate   3, **62**
Finasteride   **62**
Flagyl. See Metronidazole
Flavoxate   3, **62**

Flecainide   3, **62**
Flexeril. See Cyclobenzaprine
Floxin. See Ofloxacin
Fluconazole   3, 8, 19, 33, **63**, 108
Flucytosine   3, **63**
Flumadine. See Rimantadine
Flumazenil   **63**, **128**
Flunisolide   3, **63**
Fluoxetine   3, **64**
Fluphenazine   3, **64**
Flurbiprofen   3, **64**
Foley sizes, pediatric   **176**
Folic acid   3, **64**
Folinic acid   24, 31
Fortaz. See Ceftazidime
Foscarnet   15
Fosinopril   3, **64**, 108
Fulvicin. See Griseofulvin
Fumasorb. See Ferrous fumarate
Fumerin. See Ferrous fumarate
Fungus infection
    tinea   **30**
Furazolidone   3, **64**
Furosemide   3, **64**, 108
Furoxone. See Furazolidone

G

Gabapentin   **65**
Gamma benzene hexachloride   **72**
Ganciclovir   3, **65**
Gantanol. See Sulfamethoxazole
Gantrisin. See Sulfisoxazole
Garamycin. See Gentamicin
Gas-X. See Simethicone
Gastric lavage   **121**
Gastroenteritis   **12**
Gastrointestinal decontamination   **121**
Gemfibrozil   3, **65**
Gentamicin   3, 6, 7, 9, 10, 11, 18, 22, 23,
    25, 26, 28, 29, 32, 33, **65**, 105
    eyedrops   **105**
Geocillin. See Carbenicillin
German measles, isolation for   173
Giardiasis   **13**

Glasgow Coma Scale
  adult **135**
  pediatric **137**
Glaucoma **13**, 36, 105
Glipizide 3, **65**, 108
Glucagon 3, **65**, **128**
Glucotrol. See Glipizide
Glutethimide overdose 8
Glyburide 3, **65**, 108
Glycerin 3, **65**
Glycerol 13
Glycopyrrolate 3, **66**
GoLYTELY. See Polyethylene glycol
Gonococcal infections **13-14**, 31
Gout **14**, 174
Grifulvin. See Griseofulvin
Grisactin. See Griseofulvin
Griseofulvin 3, **30**, **66**
Guanabenz 3, **66**
Guanfacine 3, **66**, 108
Gyromitra esculenta **130**

H

H-BIG. See Hepatitis B immune globulin
Habitrol. See Nicotine transdermal
Haemophilus influenzae
  isolation for 172
  meningitis prophylaxis 19
  vaccine **175**
Halcion. See Triazolam
Haldol. See Haloperidol
Haloperidol 3, **66**
Hand
  exam **111-114**
  motor exam **112-113**
  muscle innervation **114**
  sensory nerve innervation **111**
Head injury, mannitol for **8**
Headache, migraine **14**
Heart block **147**
Heart rate, by age **177**
Height curves
  boys **181**, **183**
  girls **180**, **182**

Helicobacter pylori **9**
Hematocrit by age **177**
Hematologic indices, by age **177**
Hemocyte. See Ferrous fumarate
Hemodialysis
  for treatment of overdose **127**
Hemoglobin by age **178**
Hemoperfusion
  for treatment of overdose 127
Hemophilia A and B treatment **168-169**
Hep-B-Gammagee. See Hepatitis B
  immune globulin
Heparin 3, 21, **27**, **34**, **66**
  overdose **130**
Hepatic encephalopathy 71, 81
Hepatitis A 172
Hepatitis B
  immune globulin 3, **15**, **66**
  isolation indications 172
  prophylaxis **15**
  vaccine 3, **15**, 27, **67**, **175**
Hepatitis C
  isolation indications 172
Herpes simplex **15**
  isolation for 172
Herpes zoster 61
  isolation for 173
  treatment **34**
Hiprex. See Methenamine hippurate
Hismanal. See Astemizole
Hivid. See Zalcitabine
Homatropine eyedrops **105**
Hookworm **35**
Human bite **7**
Hydralazine 3, 9, **67**
Hydrochlorothiazide 3, **67**, 108
Hydrochlorothiazide/spironolactone 3,
  67, 108
Hydrochlorothiazide/triamterene 3, **67**
Hydrocodone/acetaminophen 3, **68**
Hydrocortisone 3, 16, **68**
Hydrodiuril. See Hydrochlorothiazide
Hydrofluoric acid, skin exposure to **122**
Hydromorphone 14

Hydroxyzine   14
Hygroton. See Chlorthalidone
Hyoscyamine   88
Hyper-Hep. See Hepatitis B immune
    globulin
Hyper-Tet. See Tetanus immune globulin
Hypertensive crisis   **15**
Hyperthyroidism   **16**
Hypothyroidism   **16**
Hytrin. See Terazosin

I

Ibuprofen   3, **68**, 108
Ilosone. See Erythromycin
Imipenem   3, 7, 21, 22, 23, 26, 28, 29, **68**
Imipramine   3, **68**
Imitrex. See Sumatriptan
Immunization schedule   **175**
Imodium. See Loperamide
Indapamide   3, **68**, 108
Inderal. See Propranolol
Indocin. See Indomethacin
Indomethacin   3, **14**, **69**, 108
Infectious diseases
    contagious periods for   **172**
    isolation periods for   **172**
Influenza   38
    isolation for   172
INH. See Isoniazid
Insulin   3, 9
Intal. See Cromolyn sodium
Intravenous drug abuse
    endocarditis   **10**
    sepsis   **29**
Intravenous fluid components   **159**
Intropin. See Dopamine
Intubation, rapid sequence   **150–151**
Iodine, Lugol's   **16**
Ipecac   **121**
Ipratropium bromide   3, **69**, 108
Ircon-FA. See Ferrous fumarate
Iron. *See also* Ferrous
    overdose   **130**, 160
Isoetharine   3, **69**

Isolation for infectious diseases   **172**
Isoniazid   3, **69**
    overdose   **130**, 160
Isopropanol poisoning   123, 127, 160
Isopropyl alcohol. *See* Isopropanol
Isoproterenol   3, **69**, 147
Isoptin. See Verapamil
Isordil. See Isosorbide dinitrate
Isosorbide dinitrate   3, **70**
Isradipine   3, **70**, 108
Isuprel. See Isoproterenol
Itraconazole   3, **70**

K

Kayexalate 3, **70**
Keflet. See Cephalexin
Keflex. See Cephalexin
Keflin. See Cephalothin
Keftab. See Cephalexin
Kefurox. See Cefuroxime
Kefzol. See Cefazolin
Keratitis, herpes simplex   **15**
Kerlone. See Betaxolol
Ketalar. See Ketamine
Ketamine   3, **70**, 150
Ketoacidosis
    alcoholic   160
    diabetic   160
Ketoconazole   3, 30, **70**
Ketoprofen   3, **71**
Ketorolac   3, 14, **71**, 108
Klonopin. See Clonazepam
Konakion. See Vitamin K
Kwell. See Lindane

L

L-Dopa. See Levodopa
Labetalol   3, **15**, **71**, 108
Lactulose   3, **71**
Lamisil. See Terbinfine
Lanoxin. See Digoxin
Laryngoscope sizes
    pediatric   **176**
Lasix. See Furosemide

Major references in **bold type**
Proprietary drug names in *italic type*
195

Laudanum 3, **84**
Length
  boys **181**
  girls **180**
Levodopa 71
Levodopa/carbidopa **71**
Levothroid. See Levothyroxine
Levothyroxine 3, **72**
Levoxine. See Levothyroxine
Librax. See Chlordiazepoxide/clidinium
Librium. See Chlordiazepoxide
Lice **16**
Lidocaine 3, **72**, 142, 144, 145, 150, 151
Lindane 3, **16**, **28**, **72**, 108
Lioresal. See Baclofen
Liothyronine 3, **72**
Lisinopril 3, **73**, 108
Lithium 3, **73**
  overdose 127
Lithobid. See Lithium
Lithonate. See Lithium
Lithotab. See Lithium
Lodine. See Etodolac
Lomefloxacin 3, 32, **73**, 108
Lomotil. See Diphenoxylate/atropine
Loniten. See Minoxidil
Loperamide 3, 12, **73**, 108
Lopid. See Gemfibrozil
Lopressor. See Metoprolol
Lorabid. See Loracarbef
Loracarbef **73**, 109
Loratadine 3
Lorazepam 3, 6, **73**
Lorelco. See Probucol
Lotensin. See Benazepril
Lotrimin. See Clotrimazole
Lovastatin 3, **74**
Loxapine 3, **74**
Loxitane. See Loxapine
Lozol. See Indapamide
Ludiomil. See Maprotiline
Luminal. See Phenobarbital
Lyme disease **16**
Lymphogranuloma venereum **17**

M
Macrobid. See Nitrofurantoin
Macrodantin. See Nitrofurantoin
Magnesium citrate 3, **74**
Magnesium sulfate 4, **6**, **9**, **74**, 142, 146
Mandelamine. See Methenamine
  mandelate
Mandol. See Cefamandole
Mannitol 4, 8, 13, **74**
Maprotiline 4, **74**
Mastitis **17**
Maxaquin. See Lomefloxacin
Maxzide. See Hydrochlorothiazide/
  triamterene
Mazicon. See Flumazenil
MCV by age 177, **178**
Measles
  isolation for 172
  vaccine 175
Mebendazole 4, **35**, **74**
Meclizine 4, **74**, 109
Meclofenamate 4, **75**
Meclomen. See Meclofenamate
Median nerve 111, 112, 113, 114
Medrol. See Methylprednisolone
Mefenamic acid 4, **75**
Mefoxin. See Cefoxitin
Mellaril. See Thioridazine
Meningitis 8, **18**
  cryptococcal **18**
  gonococcal **14**
  Lyme **17**
  prophylaxis **19**
Meningococcus
  isolation for 172
Meperidine 4, 14, **75**
Mephyton. See Vitamin K
Mepron. See Atovaquone
Mesylate. See Deferoxamine
Metabolic acidosis **160-164**
Metabolic alkalosis **161**, **162**, 164
Metaproterenol 4, **75**, 109
Methadone 4, **75**
Methanol poisoning 123, 127, **130**, 160

Methazolamide   4, **75**

Methemoglobinemia   **131**

Methenamine hippurate   4, **75**

Methenamine mandelate   4, **75**

Methenamine/phenylsalicylate/atropine/
hyoscyamine   4, **76**

Methicillin   4, 6, 7, 10, 17, 21, 22, 25, 26,
29, **76**

Methimazole   4, **76**

Methocarbamol   4, **76**

Methsuximide   4, **76**

Methychlothiazide   4, **76**

Methyldopa   4, **76**

Methylene blue   4, **77**, 131

Methylprednisolone   6, 29, **77**

Methysergide   4, **77**

Metoclopramide   4, **77**, 109

Metocurine iodide   4, **77**

Metolazone   4, **77**, 109

Metoprolol   4, 21, **77**, 109, 148

Metronidazole   4, 9, 12, 13, 17, 23, 33,
77, 109

Metubine. See Metocurine iodide

Mevacor. See Lovastatin

Mexiletine   4, **78**

Mextil. See Mexiletine

Mezlin. See Mezlocillin

Mezlocillin   4, 28, 29, 32, 33, **78**

Miconazole   4, 8, 30, 33, **78**, 109

Micronase. See Glyburide

Microsulfon. See Sulfadiazine

Midamor. See Amiloride

Midazolam   4, **78**, 150, 151

Migraine headache   **14**

Milrinone   **78**

Minipress. See Prazosin

Minitran. See Nitroglycerin

Minocin. See Minocycline

Minocycline   4, **78**

Minoxidil   4, **79**

Mintezol. See Thiabendazole

Miotic agents   105

Misoprostol   4, **79**

Mol-Iron. See Ferrous sulfate

Monistat. See Miconazole

Monocid. See Cefonicid

Monopril. See Fosinopril

Moricizine   **79**

Morphine   4, **79**

Motrin. See Ibuprofen

MS-Contin. See Morphine sulfate

MSIR. See Morphine sulfate

Mucomyst. See Acetylcysteine

Mumps
isolation for   172
vaccine   175

Mupirocin   4, **79**

Myambutol. See Ethambutol

Myasthenia gravis   **20**

Mycelex. See Clotrimazole

Mycobutin. See Rifabutin

Mycostatin. See Nystatin

Mydfrin. See Phenylephrine

Mydriacyl. See Tropicamide

Mylicon. See Simethicone

Myocardial infarction   **20**, 38

Mysoline. See Primidone

Myxedema coma   **16**

N

N-acetylcysteine. *See* Acetylcysteine

Nabumetone   4, **79**, 109

Nadolol   4, **80**, 109

Nafcil. See Nafcillin

Nafcillin   4, 6, 7, 10, 17, 25, 26, 29, **80**

Nalbuphine   4, **80**

Nalfon. See Fenoprofen

Nalidixic acid   4, **80**

Naloxone   4, **80**, 126, **131**

Naphazoline eyedrops   **105**

Naprosyn. See Naproxen

Naproxen   4, **80**, 109

Narcotic overdose   **131**

Nardil. See Phenelzine

Narrow complex tachycardia   **149**

Nasalcrom. See Cromolyn sodium

Navane. See Thiothixene

Nebcin. See Tobramycin

NebuPent. See Pentamidine
Necator americanus **35**
Nedocromil **80**, 109
Negram. See Nalidixic acid
Nembutal. See Pentobarbital
Neomycin 4, 12, **81**, 105
Neomycin/polymyxin B/hydrocortisone **81**
Neoplasm, cerebral 8
Neostigmine 4, **20**, **81**
Neptazane. See Methazolamide
Netilmicin 4, **81**
Netromycin. See Netilmicin
Neurontin. See Gabapentin
Neutropenia
  pneumonia and **26**
  sepsis and **29**
Nicardipine 4, **81**, 109
Niclocide. See Niclosamide
Niclosamide 4, **35**, **81**
Nicoderm. See Nicotine transdermal
Nicotine transdermal 4, **82**
Nicotrol. See Nicotine transdermal
Nifedipine 4, **82**, 109
Nimodipine 4, **82**
Nipride. See Nitroprusside
Nitro-Bid. See Nitroglycerin
Nitro-Dur. See Nitroglycerin
Nitrodur. See Nitroglycerin
Nitrofurantoin 4, 32, **82**
Nitrogard. See Nitroglycerin
Nitroglycerin 4, **82**
Nitroglyn. See Nitroglycerin
Nitrol. See Nitroglycerin
Nitrong. See Nitroglycerin
Nitroprusside 4, 6, **15**, **83**
  dosing chart **155**
Nitrostat. See Nitroglycerin
Nitro-Time. See Nitroglycerin
Nix. See Permethrin
Nizatidine 4, **83**, 109
Nizoral. See Ketoconazole
Nomogram
  acetaminophen overdose **125**

  acid-base **162**
  body surface area **165**
  salicylate overdose (Done
    nomgram) **124**
Norcuron. See Vecuronium
Norflex. See Orphenadrine
Norfloxacin 4, 12, 27, 32, **83**, 109
Norgesic. See Orphenadrine/aspirin
Normodyne. See Labetalol
Noroxin. See Norfloxacin
Norpace. See Disopyramide
Nortriptyline 4, **83**
Norvasc. See Amlodipine
Norzine. See Thiethylperazine
NTS. See Nitroglycerin
Nuprin. See Ibuprofen
Nuromax. See Doxacurium chloride
Nystatin 4, 8, **83**, 109

O

Odontoid process 118
Ofloxacin 4, 9, 12, 13, 32, 33, **84**
Omeprazole 4, **84**, 109
Omnipen. See Ampicillin
Ondansetron **84**
Onychomycosis **30**
Ophthaine. See Proparacaine
Ophthalmia, gonococcal **13**
Ophthalmia neonatorum **14**
Opiate
  overdose 131
  toxidrome 126
Opium tincture 4, **84**
Orchitis **12**
Organophosphate poisoning **126**, 131
Orinase. See Tolbutamide
Ornidyl. See Eflornithine
Orphenadrine 4, **85**
Orphenadrine/aspirin/caffeine 4, **85**
Orudis. See Ketoprofen
Osmitrol. See Mannitol
Osmoglyn. See Glycerin
Osmolal gap **123**
Osmolality, formula for calculated **123**

Osteomyelitis   **21-22**
Oxacillin   4, 6, 7, 10, 17, 21, 22, 25, 29, **85**, 109
Oxaprozin   4, **85**
Oxybutynin   4, **85**
Oxycodone   4, **85**
Oxycodone/acetaminophen   4, **85**
Oxycodone/aspirin   4, **86**
Oxygen
    consumption index   **157**
    content of arterial blood   **156**
    content of venous blood   **156**
    delivery index   **157**
    extraction   **157**

P

Pacemaker, cardiac   143, 146, 147
Pamelor. See Nortriptyline
Pancuronium   4, **86**
Parafon Forte. See Chlorzoxazone
Paraldehyde overdose   160
Paregoric   4, **84**
Parkinson's disease   38
Parnate. See Tranylcypromine
Paroxetine   4, **86**
Pavulon. See Pancuronium
Paxil. See Paroxetine
Peak expiratory flow
    adult   **167**
    pediatric   **166**
Pediazole. See Erythromycin/sulfisoxazole
Pelvic inflammatory disease   **22**
Penetrax. See Enoxacin
Penicillin   4, 7, 10, 16, 17, 18, 23, 24, 30, **86-87**, 109
Pentam 300. See Pentamidine
Pentamidine   4, **24**, **87**
Pentazocine   4, **87**
Pentobarbital   4, **87**
Pentothal. See Thiopental
Pentoxifylline   4, **87**
Pepcid. See Famotidine
Peptic ulcer
    treatment of H. pylori   **9**

PeptoBismol   9
Percocet. See Oxycodone/acetaminophen
Percodan. See Oxycodone/aspirin
Periactin. See Cyproheptadine
Peritonitis
    from bowel perforation   **23**
    spontaneous bacterial   **23**
Permethrin   4, **16**, **28**, **87**
Perphenazine   4, **87**
Persantine. See Dipyridamole
Pertussis
    contact management   **23**
    isolation for   172
    treatment   **23**
    vaccine   **175**
Pharyngitis   **24**
    gonococcal   **14**
    membranous   **23**
    streptococcal   **24**
Phenazopyridine   4, **87**
Phenelzine   4, **88**
Phenergan. See Promethazine
Phenobarbital   4, 6, **88**, 109
Phenobarbital/ergotamine/bella-
        donna   **88**
Phenobarbital/hyoscyamine/atro-
        pine   **88**
Phenol, skin exposure to   122
Phenothiazine overdose   **131**
Phenylbutazone   4, **88**
Phenylephrine
    eyedrops   **105**
Phenytoin   4, **88**, 109
Phosphorus, skin exposure to   122
Physostigmine   126
Phytonadione   **103**
Pilocarpine   **13**, **105**
Pindolol   4, **89**, 109
Pinworm   **35**
Piperacillin   4, 26, 28, 29, 32, 33, **89**
Piperacillin/tazobactam   7, 23, 26, 28, 32, **89**
Pipracil. See Piperacillin
Pirbuterol   4, **89**, 109

Piroxicam   4, **89**, 109
Plague, isolation for   173
Plendil. See Felodipine
Pneumocystis pneumonia
    prophylaxis   **25**
    treatment   **24**
Pneumonia   **25**
Poison Control Centers   **132**
Polio vaccine   **175**
Polycillin. See Ampicillin
Polyethylene glycol   4, **89**, **121**
Polymixin   105
Polymox. See Amoxicillin
Ponstel. See Mefenamic acid
Pralidoxime   4, **89**, 126
Pravachol. See Pravastatin
Pravastatin   5, **89**
Praziquantel   **35**, **89**
Prazosin   5, **90**, 109
Prednisone
    for pneumocystis pneumonia   **24**
Pregnancy, drug therapy in   **1**-**5**
Prilosec. See Omeprazole
Primacor. See Milrinone
Primaquine   **24**
Primaxin. See Imipenem
Primidone   5, **90**
Principen. See Ampicillin
Prinivil. See Lisinopril
Probenecid   5, 30, **90**
Probucol   5, **90**
Procainamide   5, **90**, 142, 144, 145
Procan. See Procainamide
Procardia. See Nifedipine
Prochlorperazine   5, **91**, 109
Proctitis
    gonococcal   **13**
    herpes simplex   **15**
Progesterone   9
Prolixin. See Fluphenazine
Promethazine   5, **91**
Pronestyl. See Procainamide
Propafenone   5, **91**
Proparacaine eyedrops   **105**

Propoxyphene   5, **91**, 110
Propoxyphene/acetaminophen   5, **91**
Propranolol   5, 6, 16, **91**, 110, 148
Propulsid. See Cisapride
Propylthiouracil   **16**
Proscar. See Finasteride
Prostaglandin E1   **92**
Prostaphlin. See Oxacillin
Prostatic hypertrophy, benign   62
Prostep. See Nicotine transdermal
Prostigmin. See Neostigmine
Protamine sulfate   5, **92**, **130**
Protopam. See Pralidoxime
Protostat. See Metronidazole
Proventil. See Albuterol
Prozac. See Fluoxetine
Pseudoephedrine   5, **92**, 110
Pseudogout   174
Pseudomembranous colitis   **12**
Pulmonary embolus   38
    prophylaxis   **27**
    treatment   **27**
Pulmonary vascular resistance   **156**, 158
Pulmonary wedge pressure   158
Pulseless electrical activity   **143**
Pyelonephritis   **32**-**33**
Pyrantel pamoate   5, **35**, **92**
Pyrazinamide   5, **92**
Pyrethrins/piperonyl butoxide   5, **16**, **92**
Pyridium. See Phenazopyridine
Pyridoxine   **130**
Pyrimethamine   5, **31**, **92**

Q

Questran. See Cholestyramine
Quinacrine   5, **13**, **92**
Quinaglute. See Quinidine
Quinapril   5, **93**, 110
Quinidex. See Quinidine
Quinidine   5, **93**
    overdose   **131**
Quinine   5, **93**

Major references in **bold type**
Proprietary drug names in *italic type*

R

Rabies
immune globulin **27**, **93**, 140
isolation for 173
prevention **27**, **140**
vaccine **27**, **93**, 140
Raccoon bite **7**
Radial nerve 111, 114
Ramipril 5, **94**, 110
Ranitidine 5, **94**, 110
Rape **27**
Rapid sequence intubation 70, 78, 103, **150-151**
Rat bite **7**
Recombivax HB. *See* Hepatitis B vaccine
Reglan. *See* Metoclopramide
Relafen. *See* Nabumetone
Renal failure, acute **164**
Respiratory rate, by age **177**
Retrovir. *See* Zidovudine
Reye syndrome **8**
Rheumatoid arthritis 174
Ribavirin 5, **94**
RID. *See* Pyrethrins with piperonyl butoxide
Rifabutin **94**
Rifadin. *See* Rifampin
Rifampin 5, 18, 19, 21, 22, **94**
Rimantadine 5, **94**
RMS. *See* Morphine sulfate
Roampicillin. *See* Ampicillin
Robaxin. *See* Methocarbamol
Robimycin. *See* Erythromycin
Robinul. *See* Glycopyrrolate
Rocephin. *See* Ceftriaxone
Romazicon. *See* Flumazenil
Ronase. *See* Tolazamide
Roundworm **35**
Roxanol. *See* Morphine sulfate
Roxicodone. *See* Oxycodone
Roxilox. *See* Oxycodone/acetaminophen
Roxiprin. *See* Oxycodone/aspirin
Rubella
isolation for 173

vaccine **175**
Rubeola
isolation for 172
Rythmol. *See* Propafenone

S

Salicylate overdose 127, 160
Done nomogram for **124**
Salmonella infection **12**
isolation for 173
Salsalate 5, **95**
Sansert. *See* Methysergide
Scabies **28**
Scopolamine 5, 88, **95**, 110
Sectral. *See* Acebutolol
Seffin. *See* Cephalothin
Seizures 160
Seldane. *See* Terfenadine
Selenium sulfide 5, 30, **95**
Sellick's maneuver 151
Selsun. *See* Selenium sulfide
Sensory exam
dermatomes 115, **116**, **117**
Sepsis **28**
Septic arthritis 174
Septic bursitis **7**
Septra. *See* Trimethoprim/ sulfamethoxazole
Sertraline 5, **95**
Sexual assault **27**
Shigella infection **12**
isolation for 173
Shunt **157**
Silvadene. *See* Silver sulfadiazine
Silver sulfadiazine **95**, 110
Simethicone 5, **95**
Simron. *See* Ferrous gluconate
Simvastatin 5, **95**
Sinemet. *See* Levodopa/carbidopa
Sinequan. *See* Doxepin
Sinusitis **29**
Skin infection, fungal **30**
Skunk bite **7**
Slow Fe. *See* Ferrous sulfate

Sodium bicarbonate. *See* Bicarbonate
Sodium polystyrene sulfonate 5, **95**
Sodium thiosulfate **129**
Solfoton. See Phenobarbital
Solu-Cortef. See Hydrocortisone
Solu-Medrol. See Methylprednisolone
Soma. See Carisoprodol
Sorbitol **121**
Sorbitrate. See Isosorbide dinitrate
Sotalol 5, **95**
Spectinomycin 5, 13, 14, **95**
Spinal cord levels **115**
Spinal injury
    cervical **118-119**
    cord, acute **29**
    levels sensory and motor **115**
Spironolactone 5, **67**, **96**, 110
Sporanox. See Itraconazole
Stadol. See Butorphanol
Staphcillin. See Methicillin
Staphylococcus 173
Stelazine. See Trifluoperazine
Streptase. See Streptokinase
Streptococcal
    infection, isolation for 173
    pharyngitis **24**
Streptokinase 5, **20**, **34**, **96**
Stroke 8
Subarachnoid hemorrhage 82
Sublimaze. See Fentanyl
Succinylcholine 5, **96**, 151
Sucralfate 5, **96**, 110
Sudafed. See Psuedoephedrine
Sulfacetamide eyedrops **105**
Sulfadiazine 5, **31**, **96**
Sulfadiazine, silver 5, **95**
Sulfadoxine/pyrimethamine 5, **96**
Sulfamethoxazole 5, **97**, 110
Sulfasalazine 5, **97**
Sulfisoxazole 5, 9, 19, **97**, 110
Sulindac 5, **97**, 110
Sumatriptan 5, **14**, **97**
Supraventricular tachycardia 144, **149**
Suprax. See Cefixime

Surface area nomogram **165**
Symmetrel. See Amantidine
Sympathomimetic toxidrome **126**
Synovial fluid **174**
Synthroid. See Levothyroxine
Syphilis **30**
Systemic vascular resistance **156**, 158

T

Tachycardia
    narrow complex **149**
    ventricular. See Ventricular
        tachycardia
Tacrine **97**
Taenia
    saginata **35**
    solium **35**
Tagamet. See Cimetidine
Talwin. See Pentazocine
Tambocor. See Flecainide
Tapazole. See Methimazole
Tapeworm
    beef **35**
    dog **35**
    pork **35**
Tazicef. See Ceftazidime
Tazidime. See Ceftazidime
Teeth, numbering scheme of **111**
Tegopen. See Cloxacillin
Tegretol. See Carbamazepine
Tenormin. See Atenolol
Tensilon test **20**
Terazol. See Terconazole
Terazosin 5, **97**
Terbinafine 5, **97**
Terbutaline 5, **98**, 110
Terconazole 5, 33, **98**, 110
Terfenadine 5, **98**, 110
Tetanus
    immune globulin 5, **98**, **133**
    immunization **175**
    prevention **133**, 139
    toxoid 5, **133**
Tetracaine eyedrops **105**

Major references in **bold type**
Proprietary drug names in *italic type*

Tetracycline   5, 7, 9, 16, 30, 31, **99**
Theophylline overdose   127
Thiabendazole   5, **99**
Thiamine   6, **99**
Thiethylperazine   5, **99**
Thiopental   **99**, 150, 151
Thioridazine   5, **99**
Thiothixene   5, **99**
Thorazine. See Chlorpromazine
Thrush   **8**
Thyroid storm   **16**
Thyroxine   **16**
Ticar. See Ticarcillin
Ticarcillin   5, 26, 28, 29, 32, 33, **99**
Ticarcillin/clavulanate   5, 7, 12, 21, 22, 23, 26, 28, **100**
Ticlopidine   **100**
Tigan. See Trimethobenzamide
Tilade. See Nedocromil
Timentin. See Ticarcillin clavulanate
Timolol   5, 13, **100**, 110
    eyedrops   **105**
Tinea
    capitis   **30**
    corporis   **30**
    cruris   **30**
    pedis   **30**
    unguium   **30**
    versicolor   **30**
Tioconazole   5, 33, **100**, 110
Tissue plasminogen activator (t-PA)   **20**
Tobramycin   5, 6, 7, 9, 10, 23, 25, 26, 28, 29, 33, **100**
Tocainide   5, **100**
Tofranil. See Imipramine
Tolazamide   5, **100**
Tolbutamide   5, **101**
Tolectin. See Tolmetin
Tolinase. See Tolazamide
Tolmetin   5, **101**
Tonocard. See Tocainide
Toprol XL. See Metoprolol
Toradol. See Ketorolac
Torecan. See Thiethylperazine

Tornalate. See Bitolterol
Totacillin. See Ampicillin
Toxoplasmosis
    prophylaxis   **31**
    treatment   **31**
Tracrium. See Atracurium
Tranylcypromine   5, **101**
Trandate. See Labetalol
Transderm Scop. See Scopalamine
Transderm-Nitro. See Nitroglycerin
Tranxene. See Clorazepate
Trauma score
    adult   **134**
    pediatric   **136**
Trecator-SC. See Ethionamide
Trental. See Pentoxyfylline
Triamcinolone   5, **101**, 110
Triamterene   5, 67, **101**
Triazolam   5, **101**
Trichomonas   **33**
Trichuris trichiura   **35**
Tricyclic antidepressant
    treatment   **129**
        protocol   123
Tridione. See Trimethadione
Trifluoperazine   5, **101**
Trifluridine   **15**
Trilafon. See Perphenazine
Trimethadione   5, **101**
Trimethobenzamide   5, **102**, 110
Trimethoprim   5, 24, 32, **102**, 110
Trimethoprim/sulfa   5, 9, 12, 18, 23, 24, 25, 26, 27, 29, 32, **102**, 110
Trimetrexate   **102**
Trimpex. See Trimethoprim
Trobicin. See Spectinomycin
Tropicamide
    eyedrops   **105**
Tube sizes
    pediatric   **176**
Tuberculosis
    arthritis   174
    isolation for   173
Tylenol. See Acetaminophen

Tylenol #1, #2, #3, #4. See Tylenol/codeine
Tylox. See Oxycodone/acetaminophen

U

Ulcer, duodenal **9**
Ulnar nerve 111, 114
Ultracef. See Cefadroxil
Unasyn. See Ampicillin/sulbactam
Unipen. See Nafcillin
Urecholine. See Bethanecol
Urethritis **31**
   gonococcal **13**
Urex. See Methenamine hippurate
Urinary tract infection **32-33**
Urised. See Methenamine/
     phenylsalicylate
Urispas. See Flavoxate
Urokinase **34**, 171

V

Vagal maneuvers 149
Vaginal bleeding, dysfunctional **9**
Vaginitis **33**
Vaginosis, bacterial **33**
Vagistat. See Tioconazole
Valium. See Diazepam
Valproic acid 5, **102**
Vanceril. See Beclomethasone
Vancocin. See Vancomycin
Vancomycin 5, 6, 7, 10, 11, 12, 17, 18, 19,
   21, 22, 25, 26, 29, **103**
Vantin. See Cefpodoxime
Varicella
   isolation for 173
   treatment **34**
Vascor. See Bepridil
Vascular resistance
   arterial **156**
   pulmonary **156**, 158
   systemic 158
Vasotec. See Enalapril
Vecuronium 5, **103**, 150, 151
Velosef. See Cephradine
Venous blood gases **164**

Venous pressure, central **158**
Venous thrombosis **34**
Ventricular fibrillation **141-142**
Ventricular tachycardia **141-142**, 144,
   145, 146
Verapamil 5, **103**, 110, 148, 149
Verelan. See Verapamil
Vermox. See Mebendazole
Versed. See Midazolam
Vertigo 74
Vibramycin. See Doxycycline
Vicodin. See Hydrocodone/acetami-
    nophen
Videx. See Didanosine
Virazole. See Ribavirin
Visken. See Pindolol
Vital signs by age **177**
Vitamin K 5, **103**, 129
Voltaren. See Diclofenac
Von Willebrand's disease **170**

W

Warfarin 5, **104**
Weight curve
   boys **181, 183**
   girls **180, 182**
Wernicke's encephalophathy 99
Whipworm **35**
White blood count by age **177**
Whooping cough **23**
Wounds, tetanus prophylaxis of **133**
Wyamycin. See Erythromycin
Wygesic. See Propoxyphene/acetami-
    nophen
Wymox. See Amoxicillin
Wytensin. See Guanabenz

X, Y, Z

Xanax. See Alprazolam
Xylocaine. See Lidocaine
Yersiniosis, isolation for 173
Zalcitabine 5, **104**
Zantac. See Ranitidine
Zarontin. See Ethosuximide

Zaroxolyn. See Metolazone
Zebeta. See Bisoprolol
Zefazone. See Cefmetazole
Zestril. See Lisinopril
Zidovudine   5, **104**, 110
Zinacef. See Cefuroxime
Zithromax. See Azithromycin
Zocor. See Simvastatin
Zofran. See Ondansetron
Zoloft. See Sertraline
Zolpidem   **104**
Zoster   **34**, 173
Zosyn. See Piperacillin/tazobactam
Zovirax. See Acyclovir
Zyloprim. See Allopurinol

Order form for Handbook

(3rd edition)

Please send me:

_____ copies of the *Detroit Receiving Hospital Emergency Medicine Handbook,* each $10.95 including shipping

Subtotal _____

Michigan residents add 6% sales tax _____

Total _____

Ship to:

_____

Name

_____

Address

_____

City/State/Zip

Checks payable to:
Med Center Emergency Services, P.C.

Enclose order form with payment and send to:
Handbook
Emergency Department
Detroit Receiving Hospital
4201 St. Antoine
Detroit, MI 48201

Inquiries: 313 993-2531

Order form for Handbook
(3rd edition)

Please send me:

_____ copies of the *Detroit Receiving Hospital Emergency Medicine Handbook,* each $10.95 including shipping

Subtotal _____

Michigan residents add 6% sales tax _____

Total _____

Ship to:

_____

Name

_____

Address

_____

City/State/Zip

Checks payable to:
Med Center Emergency Services, P.C.

Enclose order form with payment and send to:
Handbook
Emergency Department
Detroit Receiving Hospital
4201 St. Antoine
Detroit, MI 48201

Inquiries: 313 993-2531

8 4 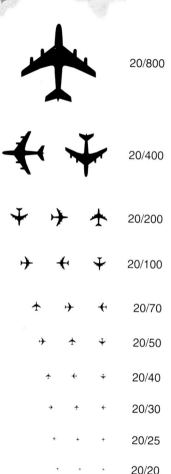 20/800

5 9 20/400

7 3 6 2 20/200

8 2 4 6 7 20/100

6 7 5 3 9 4 20/70

2 6 4 8 5 3 20/50

5 7 8 3 6 9 20/40

8 3 2 5 9 4 20/30

3 4 5 7 6 8 20/25

9 3 7 4 2 6 20/20

For visual acuity test hold 14 inches from eye